TAKE
A DEEP
BREATH

A SIMPLE EXERCISE GUIDE TO
INCREASING YOUR OXYGEN INTAKE

MEERA PATRICIA KERR
SANDRA A. McLANAHAN, MD

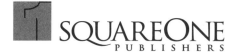

SQUAREONE
PUBLISHERS

COVER DESIGNER: Jeannie Rosado
TYPESETTER: Gary A. Rosenberg
EDITOR: Erica Shur

Square One Publishers
115 Herricks Road
Garden City Park, NY 11040
(516) 535-2010 • (877) 900-BOOK
www.squareonepublishers.com

Library of Congress Cataloging-in-Publication Data
Names: Kerr, Meera Patricia, author. | McLanahan, Sandra A., author.
Title: Take a deep breath : a simple exercise guide to increasing your
    oxygen intake / by Meera Patricia Kerr, Sandra A. McLanahan, MD.
Description: First edition. | Garden City Park, New York : Square One
    Publishers, [2020] | Includes index.
Identifiers: LCCN 2020003123 | ISBN 9780757004810 (paperback) |
    ISBN 9780757054815 (ebook)
Subjects: LCSH: Respiration—Regulation. | Breathing exercises—Therapeutic use.
Classification: LCC QP123 .K47 2020 | DDC 612.2/1—dc23
LC record available at https://lccn.loc.gov/2020003123

Printed in the United States of America

10   9   8   7   6   5   4   3   2   1

Contents

Acknowledgments, v

Introduction, 1

PART ONE

BREATHING BASICS

1. How and Why We Breathe Oxygen, 7

2. The Challenges of Lung Disorders, 21

3. Foods, Vitamins & Herbs to Improve Lung Function, 35

4. Lifestyle & Adjunctive Treatments to Improve Breathing, 57

5. Why Breathing Exercises Work, 75

PART TWO

PHYSICAL PRACTICES

6. Beginning Your Practice, 87

7. Exercises for Breathing Challenges, 93

Flex and Point, 98	Love Your Fingers, 104
Book Feet, 99	Wrist Wrangling, 105
Ankle Circles, 100	Figure Eights, 106
Knee Bends, 101	Elbow Bends, 107
Hip Juicifier, 102	Thoracic Toning, 108
Shoulder Squeeze, 103	Side Stretch, 109

Side Twist, 110

Pelvic Tilt, 111

Scarecrow, 112

Chin Up, Chin Down, 113

Side to Side, 114

Ear to Shoulder, 115

The Finale, 116

Sun Salute at the Wall, 119

Sun Salute at the Chair, 127

Torso Opener, 140

Heart Opener, 141

Hip Elevation, 142

Leg Elevation, 143

Dead to the World, 145

8. Breathing Techniques, 147

Diaphragmatic Breath, 148

Bellows Breath, 150

Alternate Nostril
Breath, 152

Humming Bee Breath, 154

Cooling Breath, 155

Wheezing Breath, 156

Hissing Breath, 157

So Hum Meditation, 159

Mantra Meditation, 161

Progressive Deep
Relaxation, 164

Conclusion, 171

Resources, 173

About the Authors, 175

Index, 177

Acknowledgments

Thank you to Dr. Amrita Sandra McLanahan for her incredible knowledge and skill in articulating the most esoteric and befuddling medical aspects of breathing and its challenges.

I must also thank publisher Rudy Shur, whose gentle urging made this book happen, with assistance from editor Erica Shur, and art director Jeannie Rosado. Thanks also to DeVries Photography studio for their expertise and good cheer.

With great love and respect, I humbly thank the tradition of yoga teachers and students who have maintained the practices of pranayama over millennia so that modern medical scrutiny can now prove the efficacy of *Take a Deep Breath*.

–MPK

With great gratitude to Rudy Shur and everyone at Square One Publishing; Dr. Gerald and Rev. Janey Lemole, my Guardian Angels on earth.

I must also thank my sister Martha Bajwa for her infinite support and encouragement, and to Gurnam Bajwa and all of the other McLanahans, and everyone at Yogaville, Virginia; Drs Robert Painter and Dwight McKee, Saraswati Newman, Montina Shraddha Cole and Shireen Lewis, of Sister Mentors, Washington, D.C., and Vimala Nora Pozzi of theIntegral Yoga Center, Richmond, Virginia.

In addition, thank you to all of my patients and friends, in the hopes we can remind each other to take deep breaths as we live more fully right here, right now, where love is always present.

–SM

To my faithful students,
who breathe life into my own practice.

MPK

To my Revered Yoga Teacher,
Sri Swami Satchidananda.

SM

Introduction

If you've picked up this book to read, it is likely that you or someone close to you is having a breathing problem. Most of us take the act of breathing for granted. Inhale, exhale . . . what could be easier? However, when the simple act of taking air in becomes noticeable, we know that something is wrong.

Perhaps it's a shortness of breath, a reoccurring cough, or a constant pain in our chest. While the symptoms and causes may vary, the bottom line is the same. Your body is not getting enough oxygen. Your lungs are no longer working to their full capacity. Hopefully, you have gone to your doctor and now have a clear idea of what the underlying issue is. The trouble is that what they have identified as the cause is not necessarily easy to fix. You were given medications to ease some of the symptoms, but were told that the problem is simply not going away.

For most people who go through this process, the prognosis is very difficult to hear. The treatments are limited and in many cases come with side effects. What you are not told is that there are a number of alternative approaches that can help to ease, relieve, or perhaps reverse your condition. Some of these approaches are relatively new; others are thousands of years old. And as you will read, all of these approaches have been found to work. Of course each condition may be different so the result can vary, but the idea is to find the ones that best work for you.

There is, however, one important consideration to remember, and it is this: Once you leave the doctor's office, you will need to take on the responsibility of improving your condition. Yes, you can take the meds you have been prescribed, but by knowing what your options are for improvement, it's up to you to do what you need to do. It's not just waiting to come back for your next appointment. It's about what you are going to do from the time you leave the doctor's office till the next visit. To a great degree, it's about controlling your own fate. That's what this book is all about.

The book is divided into two parts. Part One provides the basics behind *Take a Deep Breath*. It begins by providing pertinent medical information about the lungs that may be helpful to you. Chapter One explains the structure and function of the respiratory system. In the next chapters, various lung disorders are explained, and guidance is offered on how to use natural remedies and nutritional supplements to improve your condition. In Chapter Four the effects of stress are discussed as well as several antidotes to stress, including exercise, stretching, meditation, massage, and visualization. In the next chapters, suggestions are offered on how to prevent infection, alternative therapies that may be helpful to you, and finally an encouraging chapter on why the practices offered in Part Two of the book are going to work for you so that you can *take a deep breath!*

Part Two presents breathing exercises. All these exercises are based on time-tested practices proven to increase your breathing capacity. In Chapter Six we'll offer some tips for beginning your practice—how to sit, when to practice and other helpful ideas. Then we'll offer strategies for overcoming resistance to practice. It's not enough to read this book—it's like a refreshing bottle of water in a vending machine. It won't quench your thirst until you drop in your money, pop the top, and take a swig. Ahhh, so refreshing!

Chapter Seven guides you through some basic exercises—simple chair poses to bend and stretch the body, standing poses to build strength, and restorative poses to slow you down as you tune more deeply into your breath. You'll have practices that cool you off, heat you up, calm you down and pick you up; a little something for everybody. Finally, we dive into the breathing practices themselves. These techniques have been around for thousands of years. If you're interested in lowering stress and anxiety, yoga-based breathing is your magic carpet. The culmination of all these practices is a deeper level of self-awareness, peace, and tranquility.

HOW TO USE THIS BOOK

If you're reading this book because you're interested in expanding your lung capacity naturally, you may already be practicing some form of physical exercise—that's fine. You may want to skip over some of the more physical practices that precede the breathing techniques. But if you don't have a regular exercise routine, I advise you to start at the beginning and try the exercises in the earlier chapters in Part Two. If you're more of a visual learner, you might want to have a look at my DVD—*Big Yoga Flex-Ability*. It has a 60-minute practice that includes stretches, strengthening poses, and basic breathing techniques (see page 00 for details). Nevertheless, you can begin your breathing practice right away with the easiest and most basic of all the techniques—simple three-part breath, (see page 93 for instruction). Once you get a taste for the calm vitality produced by even a short practice, you will want to learn—and do—more. My hope is that you find as much pleasure and contentment as I do in these calming practices.

The more you know about your condition and what you can do about it, the more informed decisions you can make moving forward. It's important to point out that there are absolutely no miracle cures in this book. However as you put together your own program, you will be the first to see if your condition improves—and that can make all the difference.

PART ONE

Breathing Basics

Chapter 1

How and Why We Breathe Oxygen

nhale. Exhale. Inhale. Exhale. It seems so simple. We rarely think about the act of breathing when we are healthy. However, once we are faced with a difficult respiratory problem, we soon realize how important our lungs and breath really are. On average the human body can survive for sixty days without food. Without water, survival is only three to four days. However, without oxygen getting into your lungs, you have only four minutes before the cells in your brain begin to die, and perhaps ten minutes before your brain suffers irreversible brain damage leading to death. That's how critical your respiratory system is to your brain's well being—but there's more. A lack of enough oxygen can also affect every organ in your body. Any health issue that makes your breathing difficult and lowers the amount of oxygen your body receives can put you into serious risk of acute and/or chronic illness.

In this chapter, we will be looking at the act of breathing—how oxygen enters our body, what organs are involved, and how the oxygen circulates throughout every part of the body. This overall process is called *respiration*, and the way it operates is through our *respiratory system*. No matter what your health issue, in order to better understand its causes and alleviation, it is very important to know the basics of breathing and the role oxygen plays in keeping us healthy. As you will see, no organ in the body functions alone. They all communicate constantly, which is one reason the right breathing exercises can be so helpful for any breathing-related problems, not just with the lungs themselves, but with your overall health and well-being. By having a clear idea of what's going on in your body, you will be in a better position to choose the best options of healing for yourself.

THE ACT OF BREATHING

The action of breathing is involuntary. We do it without thinking about it. The act of drawing in air into our lungs is affected by sensors in your brain. Located in its pons and medulla oblongata regions, these specialized cells constantly measure the amount of oxygen and carbon dioxide in your blood. They tell your lungs to take in air and then release carbon dioxide. Once air enters your lungs, it moves across the membrane of the smallest sacs called alveoli—that make up the structure of the lung tissue proper—and becomes carried by the red blood cells flowing through your bloodstream. Your heart, acting as a pump, then pushes this newly oxygenated blood through to all the parts of your body, feeding them the life sustaining oxygen they all require. In summary, the respiratory system, illustrated on page 9, is thus responsible for loading the blood with oxygen, while the heart takes the job of circulating this oxygen-rich blood to the tissues, in exchange for their waste product, carbon dioxide.

As the red blood cells now carrying the carbon dioxide flow back through the lungs, the red cells there release its carbon dioxide load and next our lungs expel this waste product when we exhale. The cycle is then repeated over and over—from the moment we are born to the last breath we take. For adults this process occurs about 12 to 20 times per minute or between 17,000 to 30,000 times a day.

IT BEGINS WITH OXYGEN

When you breathe in air, you are breathing in a number of gases of which air is composed. Approximately 78 percent is nitrogen, 21 percent is oxygen, and the small remaining gases are a mix of other trace gases, such as argon, water vapor, helium, hydrogen, methane, carbon dioxide, and ozone. Of course, where you live also determines the types of pollutants that may be part of your local environment.

It is the oxygen in the air, however, that is called the "universal currency" of the body. Every cell "spends" oxygen to produce the energy it needs to do its work. When you are doing "cardio" exercising, you take in more oxygen, but you are using it up quickly for your muscles' needs. In contrast, when doing breathing exercises, the body is relatively still—so you are metaphorically putting "money in the bank."

Since the central function of the respiratory system is to exchange the major gases—taking in oxygen and releasing carbon dioxide—optimum breathing is critical. The oxygen delivered into the bloodstream and then to the red cells, is changed into the gas carbon dioxide, the waste product of cell metabolism made from this oxygen. Subsequently, this carbon dioxide gas is then eliminated from the body. When you think about it, it is both a wonder of nature and an inspiring act of life. Yes, go ahead, take as deep a breath as you can right now.

One of the first actions that is performed if you have major health difficulties, is to place an oxygen mask or prongs in your nose, so that oxygen at higher concentrations than is in regular air can be directly delivered into your lungs. The body then does not have to work as hard to make certain that oxygen gets absorbed and delivered where needed. When using this type of equipment, the percentage of oxygen can be adjusted up to 100 percent.

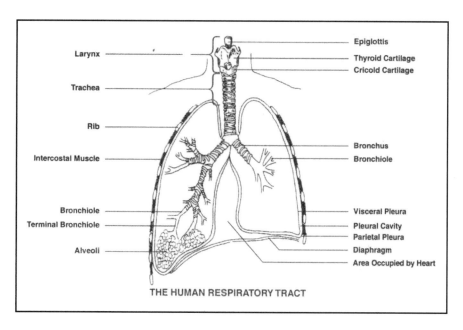

THE HUMAN RESPIRATORY TRACT

Figure 1.1. The Respiratory Tract

THE BRAIN

As we mentioned, respiration begins in the brain. Centers located in the areas called the pons and medulla, are sensitive to the amounts of oxygen and carbon dioxide in the bloodstream, and adjust your breathing rate and depth to maintain optimum levels. These control areas are in the lower portion of the brain sometimes called "reptilian," since reptiles have similar structures. If they are damaged by a stroke or accident, breathing can be completely or dangerously impaired.

While our breathing is automatic, governed by these lower brainstem centers, it is also voluntary, controlled by higher centers of thought-activated muscular contraction. You can voluntarily take a breath whenever you want to, but if your blood oxygen levels get too low, or your carbon dioxide levels too high, your brain will act to make you take a breath. You can optimize the function of both voluntary and involuntary mechanisms by doing breathing exercises to allow the best blood flow for the brain's automatic monitoring system, and for you to become more conscious of your breathing patterns. When you practice breathing exercises every day, you can train yourself to become aware to make your usual breathing slow, relaxed, and deep. As we will explore in this book, you can then affect not only your overall health, but also your sense of relaxation, joy of life, and daily inspiration with every breath.

Inspiration

We associate inspiration with things that are uplifting. The chest itself is lifted up as we breathe in, and this can be an important metaphor for life. The word for "breath" is the same as that for "spirit" in some languages, while the word "lung" means "light." The ancients put a key emphasis on breathing practices as a means to prepare the body and mind for deeper states of meditation, and ultimately, enlightenment, where the basic questions of human life are considered, "Who are we?" and "What are we supposed to be doing here?" are solved by experiencing the answers from within, from the inside out. The slow, deep breathing of the exercises given in this book can change your physiology. Breath then becomes a touchstone, allowing us to understand and experience the stillness of an unchanging reality behind our challenging, so often stressful, roller coaster lives.

The Central Nervous System

Our central nervous system consists of the brain and spinal cord. They act to provide sensation and movements. In addition, a set of nerves making up the "autonomic or automatic nervous system" are located alongside the spinal column. The portion alongside the thoracolumbar region of the middle of your back—the chest and beginning part of the low back, called T1-T12, and L1-L2—is called the "sympathetic nervous system." It activates our "freeze, fight, or flight" by causing adrenaline to be released from the adrenal glands which sit on top of the kidneys. The area of nerves in the neck and low back, called the "parasympathetic nervous system" acts to calm and relax us. The biggest parasympathetic nerve, called the "vagus," gets its name from the meaning "to wander." It meanders through the body, acting on many organs to achieve the "relaxation response" whenever it is stimulated. One way the breathing exercises work their magic is through their effects on balancing these two essential portions of our nervous system.

THE MOUTH AND NASAL PASSAGES

Breath is so important in keeping our bodies alive that we have two passageways to get air into our lungs: the mouth and the nose. The optimum way to breathe is through the nose. We *can* do it with the mouth, but breathing through the nose has special advantages. The nasal passages and sinus cavities moisturize and warm the air we breathe in, as well as trap and remove any particles, bugs, or pollen, keeping the lungs safe from colder air and invaders. This is why we have a layer of moist lining tissue in our noses: it's snot (sorry for the pun) to just give income to Kleenex tissues, and annoyance to us, but this mucus serves important immune safety functions. It traps the bad guys, so you can honk them out before they do damage. Remember this the next time you need to blow your nose. Be gentle, but don't hesitate to hoot away!

Hair and Cilia

Hair in the nose, and very small filaments lining the respiratory tract, called cilia, serve to stop particles or microorganisms from going lower into your lungs, where they can cause damage or infection. Your nasal hairs grow longer as you age, due to their lifetime exposure to the hormone testosterone, which increases their growth. Both men and women make testosterone in the adrenals; but men make more, so their nasal hairs are often especially more prominent as they age. Since they serve a protective function, don't trim your nasal hairs too short. Ear hairs protect the ear canals in a similar fashion.

Problems in the nose or sinuses, of course, arise when harmful viruses or bacteria proliferate, or an allergy develops. By increasing circulation, the breathing exercises given in this book, along with the dietary advice, can help keep your nasal and sinus passages open and healthy via improving your body's ability to do local maintenance. Cigarette, cigar smoke, and even "vape" cause paralysis of these small hair-like projections lining the respiratory tract, the cilia, so they cannot serve their function of moving trapped elements up and out of the passages. This effect is one of the reasons for chronic "smoker's cough." Fortunately, quitting smoking allows your body to reverse these damages and return to normal. Breathing practices have also been shown to help people quit smoking—if needed, please refer to the "How to Quit Smoking" section of this book on page 31.

The Nostrils

Why do we all have a left and right nostril? Why not just one big hole? Obviously the redundancy protects us if one of them is blocked. However, there is more to it. Breathing through the right nostril activates the portion of the autonomic or automatic nervous system called the sympathetic nervous system, the section of nerves in the body that wakes us up and warms us. The left nostril is connected to the parasympathetic nervous system, including the largest parasympathetic nerve called the vagus; air passing through this nostril cools and quiets your nervous system. Your breath alternates through one nostril then the other automatically every two hours or so, and thus balances your nerves. Doing the alternate nostril breathing exercise, page 80, wakes us up and calms us at the same time, and is a remarkable tool for health and healing, as we shall see.

The Uvula

The "uvula," from the Latin, "small bunch of grapes" is a smooth fleshy structure hanging down in the back of your throat. It contains glands that secrete saliva, so that it helps moisten the air that comes in as you breathe through your mouth. In addition, it adds fluid and digestive enzymes to the food you eat, so that food can pass into your digestive tract more easily.

When touched, the uvula can trigger the gag reflex, so it prevents you from swallowing food particles that are too large. It also acts during speech, assisting in the shaping of words and stopping the sounds from being too nasal.

The Epiglottis

The epiglottis is a structure at the beginning of your esophagus that when closed, prevents food from passing into the entryway of the tubes going to the lower part of your respiratory tract, and thus getting into your lungs.

The uvula and epiglottis can be activated through breathing exercises, to help the functioning of your nervous system. Consciously contracting the back of your throat and uvula area as you breathe activates the parasympathetic nervous system, the relaxation response portion of your nerves. A special breathing technique, called "contracted glottis breathing," takes advantage of this reflex activity, as presented later in this book, page 96.

The Windpipe

Air moves when we breathe in, through either the nose or mouth, to the back of the throat, where the "pharynx," derived from the Greek word for chasm or cave, leads into the "trachea," meaning "rough artery." The trachea is a tube of cartilage that then connects to the portion of the windpipe within the lung, called the main "bronchus" from the Greek meaning windpipe. Attached in front is the "larynx" from a word meaning "upper windpipe." It is the voice box, containing the vibrating cartilages which, when the air passes through, allow us to hum, speak, and sing. The "glottis" is the upper part of the larynx.

Stop That Humming

Did you know that it is impossible to hum when you pinch closed both nostrils. This is a reflection of how much your nasal cavities contribute to your voice, and another reason to do breathing practices to help keep these areas well circulated, open and healthy.

THE LUNGS

The trachea, leading into the lungs, then passes into the main bronchus. This divides into two smaller tubes, the right bronchus and left bronchus, which go directly into the right and left lungs. Then further division takes place, into smaller tubes called bronchioles, finally leading to the smallest balloon-like sacks, like bunches of small grapes, called the alveoli.

The lungs themselves each weigh about 3 pounds; the left one has two lobes, with an indentation for where the heart sits. The right lung is made up of three lobes. The lungs are the consistency of very light sponges, and have elastic fibers that allow them to expand and contract with each breath.

The Alveoli

About 300 million alveoli are found in each lung—that's a lot of grapes! They are microscopic and quite delicate. However, when stretched out, their combined surfaces would equal the size of a football field, meaning you have a lot of surface area on which your gas exchange can take place. Alveoli are where the action happens. These sacks have very thin walls, just one cell thick, so that the oxygen and carbon dioxide can pass easily through. As one gas comes in (oxygen), the other gas, carbon dioxide, goes out.

The Diaphragm

When we breathe, the main flow of air is caused by contraction of the diaphragm, a large dome-shaped muscle separating your chest from your abdomen. As it tightens, it moves downward, until it is flat, making space for more air to come into your lungs. Your chest area becomes longer and wider. The intercostal muscles, located between the ribs, also contract, widening the chest, and to a lesser extent, your neck muscles assist this basic breathing process of expansion. The diaphragm's daily involuntary movements are controlled by your brain; this automatic action can be overridden by your conscious decision to take a deep breath.

The pressure of air within the lungs opens the alveoli, so they can complete their functions. A collapsed lung termed a "pneumothorax" can occur when a portion ruptures, due to infection or injury. Air can then leak into the space between the lung itself, and the chest wall. As a result, the normal pressure dynamics can't act to inflate and deflate, and with lack of air inside, the lung shrinks down. This is called a collapsed lung. Collapse can be to a lesser or larger extent, and therefore cause few symptoms or major problems. A "chest tube" is inserted into the space between the lungs and chest wall, to drain out the air. This device has a one-way valve to prevent air from coming back in. The body may be able to repair small leaks on its own, but larger ones may require surgery.

Stretch receptors in your lungs are activated when you breathe in. They send a signal to your brain to turn on the vagus nerve, the largest parasympathetic nerve in the body, causing all your muscles to relax. So you then exhale. This activity is called the "Hering-Breuer Reflex." It helps explain why simple deep breathing can help with any stress, especially important if you have the challenge of any lung problems. Every time you take a deep breath, you activate your "Relaxation Response," governed by the parasympathetic nervous system.

You can feel the action of this reflex quite easily. Simply take a slow deep breath. You feel better right away. It's not that you are getting more oxygen to your tissues, or more carbon dioxide out—that takes more time for increased circulation from the muscle movement to have its effects on your cells. What you feel is activation of your parasympathetic nervous system, your rest and relax tend and mend sets of nerves that allow all your muscles to relax.

Go ahead. Try it. A simple few very deep breaths are enough to really help you feel more relaxed and refreshed. Unless you are going through a tunnel or in other exceptional circumstances, deep breathing throughout the day can have a significant impact on your overall health, and greatly reduce your stress.

THE HEART

Your heart is located in the central part of your chest, cushioned by the sponginess of your lungs. The pumping action of your heart is central to the function of your respiratory system—and like your breathing, your heartbeats are also controlled by your brain. Once oxygen has been moved into your bloodstream via the lungs, it is circulated to each of your cells by the pumping action of the heart. Heart attacks, other causes of heart failure, or arrhythmias can lessen the ability of your cells to receive their vital fuel of oxygen, and if so, your respiratory rate will increase to try to compensate. The breathing exercises, and other recommendations given in this book, can help to lessen the work your

Hands-Only CPR Saves Lives

If the heart fails to beat properly or stops, Cardio-Pulmonary Resuscitation (CPR) can save lives, especially if performed within four minutes, before the brain cells start to die.

First, dial 911 for assistance. Then you can begin the newest form of CPR, called "Hands-only CPR." Just compressions of the chest, 100 to 120 hard pushes per minute, have been found to be adequate for temporarily carrying oxygen to your tissues. (You can push down in beat to the tune of "Staying Alive" by the Bee Gees). There is enough residual oxygen in the blood, plus what the movements of the chest are able to bring into the respiratory system through the mouth and nose. This approach eliminates the need to blow air into the victim's mouth.

Out-of-hospital cardiac arrests have only a 12 percent survival rate; if CPR is performed, it can jump to 46 percent. (In-hospital CPR survival is about 25 percent, because patients are sicker.) Therefore you can greatly affect a person's chances of survival if you learn to use this method of CPR to treat a cardiac arrest.

CPR on Yourself

There is something called "Self-CPR," where you can give yourself some help if you think you are having a heart problem and no assistance is available. First, dial 911. Then, cough regularly. Keeping coughing can push the blood along, as well aid in correcting any irregular heartbeats.

heart and lungs have to do. Like any muscle, the heart gets stronger when exercised. In addition, whenever we take a deep breath, we push the fluids of our body along so that the heart doesn't have to work as hard. Likewise the lungs themselves get more efficient as the muscles of taking a deep breath get stronger with use.

THE CIRCULATORY SYSTEM

In addition to the heart, the circulatory system is made up of the aorta, arteries, capillaries, veins, and the blood itself. The arteries carry the bright red freshly oxygenated blood that has returned from the lungs into the heart, and then is pumped out to all parts of your body. The blood initially goes from the heart into a larger artery called the aorta. It's an important metaphor that your body is designed so that the very first arteries branching from the aorta, goes to feed the heart itself, via the coronary arteries. We need to take care of ourselves as a priority, by following the program given in this book, before we assist others.

Arteries are made of elastic tissue, so they can absorb the increased pressure created by the beat of the heart without bursting. Take your pulse point in your wrist or neck and you can feel the pump of the heart being transferred along the artery. If you cut an artery, the blood will spurt out with each heartbeat, and it appears very bright red. The arteries form into a tree-like structure, branching into ever-smaller dimensions, until they reach the level of the capillaries, which are one cell wide. This minute size allows for optimum gas exchange to the needs of your organs and cells. The red cells in your bloodstream go through one at a time, and with close proximity to the wall; oxygen can easily move through them into the tissues and cells and carbon dioxide can be picked up.

After the capillary level, the blood moves forward into your veins. They are wider and less rubbery than your arteries, and they have one-way valves within them. Since the pressure from the heartbeat has been diminished by all of the branching of the arterial system—such as when the stream from a hose is less strong the wider you make the outlet—if you cut a vein, the blood will just ooze out. Venous blood, although still red, appears slightly bluish because it contains less oxygen. Hemo-globin, the protein molecule in the blood which carries the oxygen, contains iron, responsible for the red color. When there is less oxygen,

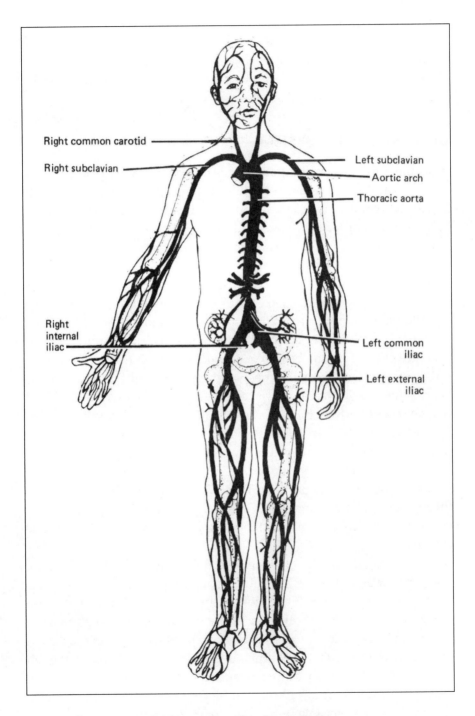

FIGURE 1.2. The Circulatory System

the diffraction of light from the hemoglobin changes the blood's color. While the pressure in the veins is lower, the one-way valves within the veins prevent blood from sloshing backwards, pulled by the forces of gravity. The blood moves along through the venous system until it returns to the heart, where the waste product carbon dioxide, a byproduct from the work of the cells that is picked up from the capillaries, can be expelled from the lungs and fresh oxygen acquired.

CONCLUSION

Our respiratory system is truly a wonder of nature. When it works properly, it can last for well over one hundred years. When it does not, it can become a major obstacle in our lives. Unfortunately, there are millions of individuals who must constantly deal with breathing issues on a daily basis. In this chapter, we have provided you with details of how our respiratory system works, and how important oxygen is to our health. In the next chapter, we will examine the most common breathing issues that infringe on our ability to be well and how the practices in this book can help alleviate problems.

Chapter 2

The Challenges of Lung Disorders

Breathing disorders can occur in two ways: (1) They can develop gradually over time. At first their symptoms may appear as a shortness of breath simply going up a staircase then later turn into difficulty breathing at rest. Or (2) they can happen quickly, based upon any number of medical issues. If you or a loved one has experienced these symptoms, you understand how life-changing such a problem can be. While some medications can temporary provide relief, the underlying causes remain, and the symptoms usually only increase. However, as you will discover, you do have some control, and there are a number of actions you can take to improve and/or stabilize your condition. The suggestions offered in this book have been scientifically proven to help you breath better.

Before we discuss these simple breathing practices and lifestyle changes that you can use in the coming chapters, it is important to first understand the specific lung disorder that is at the heart of your problem. In this chapter we will review how doctors normally test for breathing disorders and then look at the most common causes of breathing issues.

TESTING

For many centuries, physicians around the world used a simple technique to test the severity of a breathing problem. They would hold a lit candle in front of their patient and ask them to blow out the flame. The more difficult it was for a patient to blow out the candle, the more severe the problem was. As technology advanced, so did the ability of physicians to test the breathing capabilities of their patients.

Today, there are a number of tests that accurately measure respiratory function. Patients are given these tests periodically to measure the progression of breathing difficulty.

These basic tests of the respiratory function measure "cubic centimeters of air (cc)." When inflated, a six inch-sized balloon contains about 100 cc of air. The tests are performed using small measuring devices or machines into which you breathe, holding a flat nozzle in your mouth. Most common respiratory function assessments include:

- **Tidal Volume.** Measures your normal in and out breath amount: should be about 500cc

- **Residual Volume.** How much air is left in your lungs after your maximum exhalation: should be about 1,200cc

- **Inspiratory Reserve Volume.** How much more air you can breathe in after your normal inhalation: should be about 2,600cc

- **Expiratory Reserve Volume.** Amount you can breathe out after a normal exhalation: should be about 900cc

- **Vital Capacity.** Volume of air you can expel after a maximum inspiration followed by a maximum expiration: usually about 4,000cc

- **Functional Residual Capacity.** How much air remains in the lungs after a normal exhalation: should be about 2,100cc

- **Total Lung Capacity.** Amount of air in the lungs after maximum inhalation: usually 5,200cc

- **Peak Airflow.** How fast you can make the air flow; forced expiratory volume at one minute measures how much air you can forcefully blow out in one minute, and peak expiratory flow rate assesses the maximum force you can achieve.

The cause of obstruction varies with different underlying diseases. Diagnosis is made by conducting these tests of respiratory function, which focus on measuring the amount and speed of exhalation, combined with x-rays, CT scans, or MRI scans when recommended by your health care provider. Once you know what the problem is, you will have a clearer understanding of what you will need to improve your specific condition. The following section will provide you with an overview of the most common breathing disorders.

CHRONIC OBSTRUCTIVE PULMONARY DISEASE (COPD)

Chronic Obstructive Pulmonary Disease (COPD) is the overall umbrella term for chronic bronchitis, emphysema, asthma, or any other obstructing form of lung disorder when it has led to a chronic lung disorder. The most common chronic obstructive lung diseases are termed COPD and include refractory (non-reversible) chronic bronchitis, and emphysema. It is marked by shortness of breath, coughing, sputum production, and overall weakness and anxiety. What is obstructed can be at the level of the bronchial tubes, or within the alveolar sacs. Diagnosis is made through lung function tests, along with X-rays, CT scans, and magnetic imagery (MRI's).

Asthma

- Asthma is a problem of collapse or spasm of the small tubes within your lungs, the bronchi.

- Your symptoms include shortness of breath, wheezing, and difficulty breathing, especially during expiration.

- The best tests for determining if asthma is present are Forced Vital Capacity (the total maximum amount of air you can breathe in and out) and Forced Expiratory Volume (the total amount of air you can breathe out in one second).

- The breathing exercises given in this book have been scientifically shown to start right away to help with the treatment and prevention of asthma, as we shall discuss next.

Not feeling like you can exhale normally, and as if your lungs are collapsing on you, is a hallmark of asthma. You may first notice that you feel anxious, short of breath, are wheezing, coughing, or experiencing an overall sense of urgency. An increased sensation of folding in of your chest as you breathe out, points to asthma. Episodes may develop in childhood or adulthood, be brief, recurring, or ongoing, and be induced by exercise. Diagnosis is made by a combination of your health care provider listening to your chest and respiratory function tests.

The word "asthma" is derived from the Greek root "to pant." Its incidence worldwide has been increasing, probably due to more exposure to allergens and pollutants; though also keeping ourselves too clean may play a role. The "Clean Hypothesis" aims to explain why children raised on farms or around animals have less asthma—low level exposure to community bugs may prime our immune systems for protection.

Acute Asthma—One Patient's Success

Judy, one of Dr. McLanahan's patients, had gone on a weeklong vacation to the Virgin Islands. Like most holidays, it was filled with the fun of beach time, tropical breezes, and the enjoyment of a break from the usual stresses of work. However, it was also fatiguing in its own way, including the challenges of travel, adapting to the new setting, and the ambient noises. The different schedule and adjustments for family members made her feel stressed, and made sleep especially challenging. She caught a cold, and began to cough. She came back feeling tired, like she needed a vacation to recover from her vacation!

On the way travelling back, she noticed that the cough was getting worse, and that she felt a new sensation: as she breathed out, her lungs seemed to collapse in on themselves, making it harder for her to exhale. Stopping by her local physician, his stethoscope revealed that she was wheezing, and she was diagnosed with post-bronchitis induced asthma. She had previously experienced some wheezing while exercising in cold weather, but this was the first full-blown episode of asthma in her life. After the acute problem was treated, by the combination of conventional treatment and the nutritional recommendations given in Chapter 3, she began the program of breathing exercises presented in Part Two. She has never had another episode of asthma, even one associated with exercise.

Asthma can develop if your airway passages become inflamed by infection or allergic reaction, and this reaction is enough to impede airflow within your bronchial tubes, especially as you exhale. Spasm in these tubes can be induced just by anxiety; breathing exercises help to counter this tendency. Some persons are prone to asthma induced by exercise. Certain infections can be followed by a bronchitis-induced asthma. Both stress and diet have been found to be associated with this problem. In the dietary section in Chapter Three, we give recommendations for changes in foods that can be helpful, along with what supplements have been scientifically shown to make a difference.

The breathing practices given in this book have been shown by research to help reduce episodes of asthma. The authors of one study concluded: "Breathing exercises significantly decreased all component scores" of asthma symptoms. Especially useful is simply Three-Part Deep Breathing, combined with pursed-lip practice, holding the glottis as you exhale, Deep Relaxation, Meditation, and Mindfulness.

Chronic Bronchitis

- Chronic bronchitis is an inflammation of the bronchial tubes of your lungs.

- Symptoms include cough, excess phlegm, wheezing, and shortness of breath.

- Tests begin with a health practitioner listening to your lungs with a stethoscope, and the inflammation can be confirmed by chest x-ray or MRI.

- The breathing practices in this book have been documented to help in treatment and prevention, as discussed below.

"Bronchitis" means "inflammation of the bronchial tubes." If they are irritated enough, blockage can ensue. Asthma can develop.

Acute bronchitis is usually caused by infection, and treated with antibiotics when appropriate to that bug. If it is a virus-related illness, usually only supportive measure, such as fluids and rest are recommended. If you can relax during your acute episode, your body can focus on fighting the infection. Once you have recovered, you can do the program given in this book to help prevent recurrence.

If bronchitis becomes chronic, changes in diet and supplements, see Chapter Three, may be helpful. Breathing practices have also been documented to be useful. Shortness of breath was shown in one study to be diminished after only 4 weeks of practice, and lung function tests were recorded to have improved as well. Especially helpful are Three-Part Deep Breathing and Alternate Nostril Breathing, along with Deep Relaxation, Meditation, and Mindfulness.

Emphysema

- Emphysema is destruction of the basic architecture of the lungs.

- Symptoms include shortness of breath, chronic cough, and excess phlegm.

- Tests include measures of oxygen levels in your fingertip via a small device clipped to our fingertip called an "oximeter," lung function tests, chest x-rays, MRI, and blood artery tests for amount of oxygen.

- Scientific assessments have documented the benefits of the breathing exercises in this book, as we shall discuss.

Emphysema may be free of symptoms, but is usually characterized by shortness of breath. The word itself is taken from the Greek, meaning "to puff up." It is defined as a breakdown in the basic architecture of the lung, with enlarged and damaged alveolar sacs as a result. Optimum oxygen and carbon dioxide exchange is made more difficult.

Infection, smoking, pollutants, and chronic bronchitis can be at the root cause of this condition. Once the structure has been altered, it is not able to be corrected back to its original shape. However, here's where breathing practices come in. The parts that remain can get better blood and lymph supply, and other portions of the lungs *can* be opened up!

Research has shown the benefits of breathing practices for relief from the symptoms of emphysema. The most important are Three-Part Deep Breathing, Alternate Nostril Breathing, as combined with Deep Relaxation, Meditation, and Mindfulness.

Of paramount importance in preventing and treating emphysema is quitting smoking. Ninety percent of emphysema is caused by smoking. You can use the techniques given in this book to help you stop. Even one cigarette interferes with your lung function and circulation.

Please see the section on How to Stop Smoking, in the next chapter of this book. (See inset on page 31.) You can do it!

RESTRICTIVE DISORDERS

The most common restrictive lung diseases are: pneumonia and partial lung collapse. Restrictive lung problems are defined as those that reduce the total volume of your lungs, due to changes in the characteristic of your lung tissue or from diseases which affect your chest's ability to expand and contract successfully. These disorders are further divided into those that reduce the internal lung surface in which gas exchange can take place, and the ones that are extrinsic, caused by chest and neuromuscular abnormalities. The abbreviation PANT is used to summarize the causes of restrictive lung problems: it stands for pleural (the lining of the lungs), alveolar (at the level of the smallest segment of your lungs, the alveoli,) interstitial (between the tissues of the lungs), neuromuscular, (challenges with muscles or nerves) and thoracic cage abnormalities.

COPD Can Be Improved

Matthew, a patient who came to see Dr. McLanahan, had been diagnosed with COPD by respiratory testing and x-rays. He was a two-pack a day smoker, and had smoked for forty years. Even though he wanted to quit, he just had a hard time sticking to his resolve to do it. A rural farmer, now he was having more and more difficulty simply carrying out his daily chores. He was also experiencing mood changes new to him, feeling depressed and discouraged for the first time in his life. He was willing to try something different.

He began doing the breathing program and dietary changes given in this book, and found that he felt better almost immediately. He was able to finally quit smoking, and his color changed from appearing gray to a healthy glow. He also began to feel better overall, more peaceful and hopeful, and his respiratory function tests improved. Whenever he skipped his daily practice, he noticed that he felt worse. He put on music during his sessions, to encourage himself, and began to enjoy life more and more fully.

These problems are diagnosed, as with the obstructive issues, via lung function tests, along with specific tests of neuromuscular activity. Intrinsic restrictive diseases can be caused by immune diseases, such as rheumatoid arthritis, certain types of pneumonia, exposure to cigarette smoke, or chemicals in the environment. Extrinsic causes can include infections like polio-like viruses, the breakdown of your neuromuscular apparatus from diseases such as muscular dystrophy, or the effects of aging on the up-right posture of our spine.

Breathing exercises can act to strengthen your muscles, and help to treat both intrinsic and extrinsic restrictive lung disorders. One study found that for patients who have received cardiac surgery, who are at risk for restrictive lung problems associated with their pain and stitches, breathing exercises improved symptoms and shortened recovery times.

Pneumonia

- Pneumonia is infection or inflammation of the small alveolar sacs of the lungs, which fill with pus and sometimes blood, so that air can't effectively pass through them.

- Symptoms may include chest pain, shortness f breath, chills and/or fever, sweating, loss of appetite, and weakness.

- Tests include a health practitioner listening to your lungs, chest x-rays, MRI.

- The breathing exercises given in this book have been shown to help in the relief of symptoms and prevention of pneumonia, as we shall discuss.

The word pneumonia derives from the roots "pneuma" meaning "air," and referring to the lungs, and "onia" meaning "a burden." Pneumonia, in general, is an inflammation of the alveoli (air sacs) of the lungs caused by a viral, bacterial, or fungal source. These alveoli can fill with fluid, pus, or blood, making your breathing difficult. Pneumonia may be associated with few symptoms or can be accompanied by a cough (that may produce dark green or blood-tinged phlegm), fever, and chest pain. It can affect one or both lungs, and can be mild—the so-called "walking pneumonia,"—or life-threatening. Pneumonia can develop following a cold or the flu, it is more common if you become more sedentary, as you age, or if your immune system is compromised. Fortunately, the breathing exercises given in this book can help you avoid pneumonia, or strengthen you as you recover.

During the acute phase of your illness, usually lasting one to two weeks, the best approach is to rest as much as possible. You can still do some mild three-part breathing, the Deep Relaxation, and meditation practice, but generally just take it easy, drink lots of fluids, and rest, rest, rest. Then you can slowly commence the program given in Part Two of this book, beginning with the chair positions. It will help to clear any lingering cough. At first, go half as far as you are comfortable, honor your own body, and do not strain. The saying is "The easy path is hard enough," and it applies especially as you recover. Posture can affect your chances of pneumonia, so using your breathing practice to remind you to sit upright, with your shoulders back and "squared" can help make your lungs move their fluids along, to get the white cells to where they need to fight any possible infection. Make your practice fun, do it regularly, and within a short time you can start to notice its benefits. Even one session should make you feel better and ease your breathing.

After you have had one episode of pneumonia, your lung function may remain changed. One study found that increased tiredness was still present three months afterwards, for half of those affected, and one-third still had cough and shortness of breath. Having one bout can make it more likely you will have another. You can help prevent and reverse this by regularly practicing the breathing program given in the second part of this book.

Partial Lung Removal

- You may require removal of part or all of one or more lungs, due to injury or cancer.

- You may be able to live quite comfortably; Pope Francis has functioned for many years after a portion of his lung was removed. Symptoms may include shortness of breath.

- The standard lung function tests are given.

- Research supports the use of the breathing exercises in this book to improve the function of your remaining lung tissue.

If you have to undergo removal of part of your lung for some reason, you can use the breathing program given in this book to help you recover. Since you have five lobes of lung tissue, a significant amount of extra cushion to your breathing mechanism is built in. Under normal conditions, we are generally using only about 70 percent of lung tissue capability. Surgery can reduce your lung volume by quite a lot before you develop symptoms. In any case, you can optimize the function of your remaining amount of lung by doing the breathing exercises given in the second half of this book. Research with patients who survived lung cancer has documented the benefits of breathing exercises.

CONCLUSION

If you have been diagnosed with the COPD challenge, here is some heartening encouragement: the symptoms of COPD have been scientifically shown to be lessened by the breathing practices given in this book. In one research study, one hour practice daily showed improvements in all of these measures within 6 weeks.

These practices work first of all by increasing local blood and lymph circulation, so that your body can do better repair work. In addition, because they help you relax, your body can focus its resources on fixing underlying problems more effectively—blood and lymph flow changes when we relax, with improved resources for effective immune function and overall health maintenance. The scientific research has documented the positive effects of breathing practice on respiratory function by themselves. The standard lung function tests are improved within as short a time as a few weeks. In addition to noticing the effects of your practice on your symptoms, you can have these tests performed by your health care provider, and follow your progress that way. (For ways to quit smoking by using the *Take a Deep Breath Program*, see the inset starting on the following page.)

How to Quit Smoking
Using the Take a Deep Breath Program

If you smoke, the most important action you can take to reduce your chances of developing lung problems is to quit. Sounds simple. Some estimates say cigarettes are as addictive, or even more, as opioids, including heroin. Up to half of all illness in the United States could be eliminated if everyone stopped smoking. Some surgeons now even refuse to operate on smokers, since their outcomes are so much worse from any surgery. However, there is good news. A breathing exercise program can change your brain's addictive patterns, and dietary choices can make a difference in your chance of success in stopping. This book offers you much to help you quit, and stay off cigarettes for good.

- **Decide to Just Do It.** The first step in quitting is deciding to do it. Making up your mind to *Do It Now* is often all it really takes to be successful. Focusing on the bad effects of even one cigarette—which interferes with your circulation enough to lower the skin temperature in your hands and feet by two degrees (one of the reasons smokers have more wrinkles)—may help get you motivated. Pictures of the ravages of smoking, placed on the packages of cigarettes, have been found to help people quit. You can place them around where you are tempted, to remind yourself to just do it.

- **Practice the Breathing Program Given in This Book Daily.** Permanently quitting smoking, like losing excess weight and keeping it off, is often preceded by many unsuccessful skirmishes. Your addiction may have its psychological roots in oral or other nourishment issues, and let's admit it, smoking is often useful as a stress-reducing habit. Therefore, you need to have a substitute stress management program in place, to achieve the relaxation represented by the magic of the cigarette break.

That's the role of your daily breathing program. Many studies have documented the remarkable effects of these practices to help people permanently stop smoking, and you have the side benefit of improving the quality of your life as well.

- **Practice Visualization.** Circling in red the exact date you want to quit can help. Whenever you crave a cigarette, you can picture that calendar in your mind's eye, and say to yourself, "No, that's it, that's the date I quit. Never again."

- **Use Massage and Water Therapy.** Smoke-enders retreats have found that relaxation in a shower, bathtub, or hot tub to be especially soothing during the quitting process. After such a weekend at a spa, one of the staff told me that afterwards they found it necessary to drain the hot tub and scrub it down, because the tub water turned yellow from all the nicotine sweated out from the bodies of the smokers!

- **Use Hypnosis and Acupuncture.** These modalities have quite high success rates, though you may need more than one or two sessions.

- **Use Chewing Gum and Toothpicks.** Smoking is orally satisfying. Choose gum only that's sweetened with stevia—otherwise it can contribute to tooth decay and in the case of aspartame, cause depression by lowering serotonin levels. The act of chewing raises serotonin levels, which makes you feel good, and using toothpicks to push down on the gums helps them stay healthy and prevents infection. Gum disease causes chronic inflammation in the body, and increases your risk for heart and lung diseases.

- **Use Herbal Remedies.** The herbs chamomile, valerian, lavender, taken as teas, can provide soothing relief from the jagged feelings of withdrawal. Aromatherapy with lavender, rose, or jasmine essential oils sprinkled on your clothing or pillow, put in the bath or a room diffuser, or in massage oils which you can apply to yourself or ask your massage therapist to use, can help you achieve and maintain a relaxed state.

- **Use Medications.** A nicotine patch or nicotine gum may be necessary. Other drugs may be needed, but monitor their side effects.

Other Natural Adjuncts—Massage

As we have discussed, just taking a deep breath changes your physiology; your body's activity and chemistry is altered beneficially, your mind's action shifts to a more tranquil state, and you can get in touch with a quiet, peaceful center of yourself in the midst of whatever is happening in your daily life.

Therapeutic massage can also give you these kinds of benefits, as well as help you physically take easier, deeper breaths. Tight muscles prevent the fullest excursion of your breathing mechanism, and regular massage can lengthen and loosen your muscles on a regular basis. Blood and lymph fluids are moved along, so that they can more effectively perform their maintenance functions.

Benign touch itself has been shown to increase parasympathetic nervous system activity, leading both to you feeling more relaxed, and your physiology being able to tend and mend more effectively. You can try various styles of massage, or use self-massage, to see what works best for you.

Massage lowers the stress hormones adrenaline and cortisol. It can help you sleep better, so that the body can do better repair work. Massage has been shown to help with anxiety and depression, which can often accompany COPD and other lung diseases. Massage can also help with smoking cessation. Massages given to those suffering from asthma were documented to improve pulmonary function tests. In one summary study, patients receiving regular massages reported "improved health" and "less breathing difficulty" even when their lung functions tests were only minimally better.

We recommend you obtain massages as often as you can fit them in; you may also trade massages with a spouse, friend, or child, or purchase a massage chair, as well as do "self-massage." The main principles are using gentle, firm strokes, always moving towards the heart. This allows your lymph and blood to be assisted in their circulatory work.

A wide array of massage traditions are now available, which you can sample until you find what makes you feel most comfortable. These are the ones we most recommend:

- **Deep Tissue/Swedish.** Often used with oils and aromatherapy, this style allows a significant release of your muscles and movement of fluids through the deep tubes of your blood and lymph systems. The therapist's hands stroke all parts of your body, in the direction of your heart. Your muscles lengthen and loosen, and your fluids are moved along. As you relax, your breathing becomes slower and deeper. Research has shown that this type of massage can especially benefit asthma patients.

  When compared with other styles of massage, this approach exhibited more physiological change towards deeper relaxation and effectiveness. Therefore, you might want to try various therapists until you find one with which you are most comfortable.

- **Acupressure/Shiatsu.** These Asian traditions use specific points along energy pathways called meridians, to relax muscles and improve circulation. Pressure is applied to these points, which are then massaged, and sessions can vary in length. The specific points have been mapped out; you can find charts online, and give yourself a self-massage to achieve benefits. This approach can be especially helpful if you don't have time or place for the full body deeper massage. You do not need to disrobe, and sessions can take only a few minutes for you to feel the effects.

  Research on "sham" acupressure points has come to no conclusion about whether the real points make a difference. However, much research supports acupressure as a relaxing modality to be added to your daily life, whether it works via placebo pathways or not.

- **Rolfing.** This technique utilizes deep tissue re-alignments to change posture. It was first developed by a massage therapist named Ida Rolf, who observed what regular yoga practice did to the body, and wanted to accelerate these benefits via massage. Rolfing therapists use deep strokes, even sometimes using their elbows, to realign your musculo-skeletal structure. This approach can especially help those with COPD, which is commonly associated with curvature of the spine forward. Research has shown, with before and after x-rays, that scoliosis and other back postural problems can be improved. Sessions typically take 90 minutes.

Chapter 3

Foods, Vitamins & Herbs to Improve Lung Function

The health of your lungs as well as every other part of your body is affected by the foods you choose to eat. Research has shown that your dietary choices can help prevent lung disorders, along with assisting in recovery once they develop. If you already have COPD, for example, merely eating one extra serving of fresh fruits per day was documented to give a 24 percent decreased risk of dying from your disease. On the other side, ingesting cured meats, such as bacon, salami, ham, bologna, sausage, or hot dogs directly increased risk for COPD. Lung function of COPD patients was found to improve within two weeks of adding more fruits and vegetables to their diets. If you have difficulty chewing solids, consider turning them into easy-to-drink smoothies. In this chapter we will give a Superdrink smoothie recipe page 48, to help you add more fruits and vegetables to your eating plan, in blended form, on a daily basis.

The essence of the dietary recommendations in this chapter is this: eat foods that that fight inflammatory, and avoid those that cause inflame. (See inset on page 36.) Inflammation is a causative agent in many lung problems, and markedly affected by your dietary choices. A simple rule of inflammation, as we shall see in this chapter: whole foods, vegan diet lowers inflammation levels, while the usual animal food based diet raises these immune effects.

What Is Inflammation?

Inflammation is defined as the redness, swelling, heat, and pain created as a reaction within tissues of your body. It is usually due to an allergic response, or due to an injury or infection. It is part of your body's defense mechanism, a side effect of the white cells and other elements of your immune system simply doing their jobs to clear problems. Inflammatory reactions can be created by genetic sensitivity, any injury, cigarette smoke and other pollutants, chemicals, and various elements of the diet to which an individual may be sensitive.

The most common inflammatory foods are:

- Dairy products
- Sugar
- Hydrogenated oils
- White flour
- MSG
- White rice
- Saturated fats

The best anti-inflammatory foods are:

- Fresh fruits
- Ground flaxseeds
- Fresh vegetables
- Onion
- Garlic
- Oregano
- Ginger
- Turmeric

As research has shown, by avoiding the first list of food items and adding the second group of ingredients into your daily diet can make an immediate impact on your lungs.

Nutrition can help modify the effects of cigarette smoke and even help prevent lung cancer from spreading. It can diminish the thickness of your lung secretions, assisting to prevent and reverse cough, congestion, and pneumonia. For example, many people have much better lung function by just giving up all dairy products, a common source of allergy and inflammation. A plant-based diet, rich in fruits and vegetables, can not only help prevent and fight infections but also change your "epigenetics," the expression of your genetic inheritance, and lengthen the ends of your chromosomes, which affect aging. The proverbial Fountain of Youth may be as near as your fork, knife, and spoon!

The digestive system is central in your body, and its actions, that help turn broccoli, almonds, and myriad other foods into the nutrient components that feed your cells, can affect your muscle strength, immune capability, ability of your blood to circulate and carry nutritional elements, your weight and mood, and your overall function in life, quality of life, and lifespan. Yes, we are what we eat, on many levels: we now know scientifically that dietary choices make a difference. The diet high in fruits and vegetables that have been shown to slow the progression of COPD, and improve lung function, is presented in this chapter. We will give you guidance about the most optimum nutrition plan for your lung health and healing. In addition, we will try to make your lifestyle choices with regard to nutrition sustainable and fun, using substitutes for your favorite staples, so that it's easier for you to stick to it.

HOW DO YOU KNOW WHAT TO CHOOSE?

So much controversy has swirled around what constitutes the best diet, and much of this advice has been at polar opposites. Fortunately, enough research has shown the ideal trends, and even the various food camps agree on many basics. For example, it can be agreed on that raw fresh vegetables, including two bunches of dark leafy greens per day, are essential for everyone, and our need for fiber has been well established. Fiber is only found in plants, so they need to be the basic building blocks of each meal. This helps provide enough fiber for good bowel function: you need to eat sufficient fiber to have two to three bowel movements per day. Every time you relieve your bowels, it activates your parasympathetic nervous system, (PNS) the part of your nerve activity that invokes the Relaxation Response, so that all the muscles in your body relax a little. We even say that we have "relieved ourselves." There is nothing quite like a good bowel movement to make you feel like whistling!

In the last decades, the emerging science of human nutrition has shifted and grown by bounds, leaps, and curlicues. The wisdoms of many of our parents' choices have been set aside, but it looks as if, especially in the case of the advice "eat your vegetables," about some things they were right. The injunction of Hippocrates, "Let Food Be Your Medicine," is leading to new fields—dark, green, and leafy—of medical research and health maintenance.

"We dig our graves with our teeth," goes an old saying. It's not just for good lung function. What kind of diet you should be following in general has some basic principles, and your food choices help determine your risk for infection, cancer, osteoporosis, heart disease, and a smorgasbord of other physical conditions that affect lung function. Some foods are especially detrimental, while others may offer protection and even therapeutic benefit once an illness or disorder has developed.

First impressions have been found to last a bit longer. Hearing the good news first can inspire us to take on anything that is difficult. In the beginning focus on the foods you like that are good for you, avoiding the detrimental ones, and gradually introduce the foods you find yukky. Fortunately, our tastes do change. We tend to crave the foods we eat regularly, as our palate shifts. The good news in nutrition is that more and more substitutes are available for harmful items. Some old staples like oatmeal have achieved a new status, with increasingly interesting ways emerging to prepare and present healthy foods that previous generations may not have known about, which place the more painful medicinal aspects in the background.

PLANT-BASED DIETS

The aim of the breathing exercises given in this book is to prevent and reverse lung disorders, but it also assists in just making you feel better. In our culture, food is not only eaten for fuel, but often to deal with stress. The breathing program can help you experience a deeper ongoing sense of ease, increased mindfulness, love, and ability to enjoy life. Whenever you do eat something, you can enjoy it even more, and yet curb your cravings or overindulgences. The dense, saturated fats found in animal foods slow down your digestion, physically obstruct your circulation, and shift your hormones in a detrimental direction, such as causing a rise in adrenaline. In one Harvard study, persons fed beef disguised in biscuits were found to have an increase in blood pressure, LDL cholesterol, and anxiety levels.

Broccoli, kale, cabbage, Brussels sprouts, and the spices curry (containing the spice turmeric), ginger, and oregano are foods to emphasize in your diet, since they have specific immune boosting effects that not only can help fight infection, but also assist in the prevention and treatment of cancer. We will give you a list of the best foods to include weekly, along with a general guideline for meals (See page 40).

All digestion begins in the mind: stress in your mind interferes with the resources of your blood supply going to your digestive tract. Prayer or a short period of silence before meals is recommended. Vegans have been shown to be happier and healthier. This nutritional program has been documented to lower risk not only for lung disorders, but also heart disease, strokes, cancers of the skin, breast, colon, prostate, esophagus, gallbladder, and thyroid, as well as leukemia and lymphoma. In addition, lower rates of thyroid goiter, Down syndrome, Alzheimer's, and multiple sclerosis have been found.

FIBER

Fiber is defined as the portion of a plant which passes through the digestive tract without being absorbed. Fiber is only found in plants. Meats, eggs, and dairy contain no fiber. Originally sometimes called "roughage," fiber is really ore like "softage." It keeps your foods moving through your gut and helps prevent an array of diseases, especially colon and other cancers, as well as heart disease. Two main types of fiber are identified: soluble, found primarily in fruits and oatmeal; and insoluble, found mostly in vegetables and whole grains. You need both types. The soluble form traps more fats and cholesterol and removes them from your body; the insoluble one keeps your bowels moving along with optimum bulk.

Much scientific documentation suggests that a high fiber diet is essential for the health, not just of your colon but your lungs as well. If your belly is filled with food and pushing upward, less space is available for your diaphragm to contract and open up your lungs for their full complement of air. About 20 to 40 grams of dietary fiber are considered optimum. The average American takes in only five grams. As a result, we are one of the most constipated countries in the world.

Just adding oat bran to a diet low in fiber may not provide adequate protection. You want to aim at a pound to a pound of stool per day.

Super Foods to Include in Your Diet

Lots of articles and ads can be seen touting the term *super foods*. But exactly what are super foods? As a rule, they refer to whole foods that contain the most fiber, vitamins, and minerals, along with the best ratios of protein, carbohydrates, and fats for you to regularly incorporate into your diet. Try to eat some of them each week. Eating from the cruciferous family—kale, broccoli, cabbage, Brussels sprouts, bok choy—just three times a week has been found to lower your risk of cancer. We recommend the following foods, listed in order of convenience. Aim for two salads a day, 3 to 4 servings of fruits, a cup of legumes, and a cup of whole grains.

- **Fruits.** Berries and cherries, oranges, grapefruits, lemons, limes

- **Herbs and Spices.** Chives, cilantro, curry, garlic, ginger, onions, parsley, and turmeric

- **Legumes.** Beans (such as red, black, kidney beans), lentils, soy products, like soy beans (edamame), soy burgers, soy chicken, soy or tempeh bacon, soy cheese, soy milk (unsweetened)

- **Raw Salad Items.** Beets, broccoli, Brussels sprouts, cabbage, cauliflower, dark leafy greens, tomatoes

- **Seeds and Nuts.** Flaxseeds (freshly ground to cracked), raw unsalted almonds, almond milk (unsweetened), pumpkin seeds

- **Steamed Vegetables.** Any whole cooked vegetable can be included, and it is most nutritious when steamed; especially often, choose carrots, sweet potatoes

- **Whole Grains.** Brown rice, quinoa

Eliminate low fiber foods, such as those made with white flour, white rice, and refined sugar, and replace them with fresh fruits, vegetables, and whole grains.

FATS

Fats in your diet can be of varying kinds: "saturated," generally solid at room temperature; "mono-unsaturated," semi-liquid; and "unsaturated," remaining liquid. The "saturation" amount refers to the basic chemical structural form of the fat. The thicker, less flowing saturated fats obstruct and inflame the arteries and lymph channels more, helping to explain why they interfere with maintenance of your health. Fats from animal foods tend to be more saturated, and have been correlated with an increased risk for cancer, while those that come from plants are not. The total amount of fat you eat per day, regardless of saturation, has also been found to be correlated with your risk for disease.

Most Americans eat from 30 to 50 percent of their calories from fat. To prevent and treat disease, the ideal number is now felt by many researchers to be between 10 to 20 percent. You can best achieve this by eliminating animal foods and dairy. Instead use clean sources of protein not linked to a high amount of fat, such as beans, bean sprouts, lentils, green beans, green peas, dal (a small Indian quick-cooking lentil), soybeans and soy products (which do not increase risk of breast cancer or lower testosterone, as was falsely believed, but in fact decrease risk of cancer—the phytoestrogen they contain does not act like estrogen).

Saturated fats are inflammatory to your body, putting you at risk for illness. Fats are made from fatty acid components, which we can mostly manufacture in our bodies. You don't need to eat fish to get your required anti-inflammatory "omega-3" type of fat. After more than 30 years of research, no lack of essential fatty acids has been found in following patients on the Dean Ornish vegan plan for preventing and reversing heart disease, diabetes, cancer, and other diseases. The two "essential" fatty acids omega-3, DHA, and EPA, which we must eat can be obtained from adding your vegan diet; the ALA type of fatty acids found therein can be converted to DHA and EPA by your body as needed. In addition, the lower amounts of pro-inflammatory omega-6 fats in the vegan diet means that you do not require as large amounts of anti-inflammatory omega-3 in your diet, since it is the ratio of these that is felt to contribute to the deficiency of omega-3s and to the onset of disease. You can also insure adequate amounts of omega-3 in your body by eating some seaweed regularly, or take vegan capsules derived from algae, as discussed on page 52 in the supplement section of this chapter.

Make certain always to avoid the so-called "Trans-fats," listed on food labels as "hydrogenated" or "partially hydrogenated" oils. These are man-made substances that have been linked to increased free-radical (cell elements that accelerate aging) damage, and they raise the "bad cholesterol" (LDL) levels while lowering the "good cholesterol," (HDL). Cook only with small amounts of olive oil, and add only minute amounts to your salads and other foods. If you think about it, no animal in the wild adds oils to their foods. Enough natural oils are present in the foods themselves. Our closest genetic relatives, the gorillas, are all vegans, and plenty strong. The best science supports eating our foods as close as possible to how they are found in nature.

- **Best good fat foods:** Beans, lentils, green peas, and green beans

- **Worst bad fat foods:** Fried foods, hydrogenated and partially hydrogenated oils, red meats, and dairy

For those who already have heart or lung disease, these foods also need to be avoided: any added oils or oil-based dressings, mayo or even vegan mayo, avocado, nuts and nut butters, hummus, and coconut. They restrict blood flow—imagine how a greasy pipe inhibits optimum flow, and your capillaries are only one hair thick. Instead, choose foods that flow.

PROTEINS

Ingesting proteins from animal sources has been associated with increased risk for disease, especially heart problems and cancer. Protein from vegetable origins has not been found to correlate with these disorders. The particular ratio of amino acids in animal foods, compared to that of vegetables, when presented to your body's glands, creates altered hormone output which in turn is felt to account for the increased cancer rate. An excess of animal protein has also been correlated with chronic kidney disease. In any case, a plant-based diet can help you avoid not just lung disease, but other problems that can impact your lungs' ability to function optimally.

The best plant based sources of protein include peas, beans, green beans, lentils, dal, and soy products, such as tofu and tempeh, along with raw nuts and seeds (no more than a handful per day, since they are high in calories, and keep them in the fridge to prevent them from becoming rancid). Beans contain more protein per pound than beef! We do need to ingest certain "essential" amino acids, the components of proteins, from our diets. However, you can get all the essential amino acids you need by combining beans and grains. You do not have to do it as at every meal; the liver stores amino acids over weeks. While 35 to 50 grams of protein per day are adequate for for most people, very active persons and pregnant women may need as much as 100 grams per day.

- **Best High Proteins Foods:** Beans, green peas, green beans, lentils, and soy products

PHYTOCHEMICALS

Phytochemicals are natural constituents of plants and fruits that provide particular benefits to your immune system and hormone levels. For example, lycopene, a substance found in higher amounts in tomatoes, pink grapefruits, and watermelons, is a powerful antioxidant (a substance that fights aging) with proven ability to help prevent cancer. More than a hundred phytochemicals have been differentiated and implicated in helping prevent disease. The best way to assure your adequate intake of these vital substances is to frequently include berries, citrus fruits, tomatoes, cruciferous and dark green leafy vegetable, whole grains, seeds, and beans in your diet, along with onions, garlic, and cayenne pepper.

- **Foods highest in antioxidants:** Artichokes, beets, berries, kale, red cabbage, spinach, watercress, as well as black, kidney, and red beans,

- **Foods highest in lycopene:** Asparagus, tomato sauce, red cabbage, red grapefruit, and watermelon

- **Foods highest in anthocyanins and other helpful phytonutrients:** Beets, black rice, blackberries, blueberries, dark cherries, pomegranates, purple grapes, purple plums, and red cabbage

REFINED SUGAR

Up to 80 percent of foods sold in supermarkets contain refined sugar, a habit-forming component. This refined sugar is an ingredient added to infant formulas and many baby foods, producing a taste attraction at an early age that may last way into adulthood.

You Are Sweet Enough:
The Dangers of Refined Sugars

Refined sugar is an addictive ingredient added to up to 80 percent of foods found in supermarkets. Especially vulnerable to such inducements are children, when it is added to infant formulas, baby foods, and cereals, creating a taste incentive from the beginning of our lives. Even in the womb, your tastes can be shaped by your mother's dietary choices, making it harder for you to control your sweet teeth when they emerge.

Regular ingestion of refined sugar has been associated with the development of some cancers, as well as with heart disease, diabetes, and obesity in general. Finding a replacement can impact your lung health by improving your immune system function. Even one tablespoon of refined sugar has been shown to lower the activity of your white cells to fight infections, and prevent diseases, such as heart disease, diabetes, and cancer. A 60-percent higher refined sugar intake was found in women who developed breast cancer. Diabetics have more vascular and circulatory problems, affecting their lung's ability to do repair work. Even if you are not diabetic, when your blood sugar is pushed up after eating that beckoning dessert, your white cells are less capable of keeping you safe: their immune surveillance is sabotaged. Eating sugar also increases risk for gum disease, which increases inflammation in your body and puts you at higher risk for heart and lung disorders.

The sugar content of a product may be hard to find simply by reading the ingredients label. A multitude of other names mask its total presence. For example, maltose, glucose, dextrose, maltodextrin, brown rice syrup are code names, but they still have detrimental effects on your blood sugar and thus your immune system. In general, eat whole fresh foods, rather than those from a package, and avoid those with any added sweeteners, even honey. When baking, use bananas or apples to add sweetness.

Consuming refined sugar on a daily basis has been linked to the growth of some cancers, in addition to other diseases, such as heart disease, diabetes, and obesity. Eliminating or replacing this ingredient in your foods can also improve your immune system function and your lung health. Women who were diagnosed with breast cancer showed a 60 percent higher consumption of refined sugar. A diet that includes refined sugar also creates vascular and circulatory issues, especially for a diabetic, acting on their lung's ability to repair.

Your blood sugar level rises, even if you are not diabetic, when you allow yourself to be enticed by the decadent dessert; white cells become less active to fight infection and remove cancerous cells. As little as one tablespoon of refined sugar has been found to interfere with this maintenance action of your blood's white cells, sabotaging the multiplication of cancer cells. Gum disease, which increases the risk of inflammation in your body and puts you at a higher likelihood for heart and lung disorders, is also linked to the consumption of refined sugar.

- **Best foods to satisfy your need for sweets:** Fresh whole fruits, the spices cardamom, and cinnamon.

ALCOHOL

Staying away from alcohol can help your daily lung function, as well as assist in preventing many diseases in the long run. Drinking alcohol regularly has been scientifically documented to increase your risk for COPD, probably due to its detrimental effects on the immune system. Alcohol raises blood sugar levels, which influences your white cells to be less active. They can't do their maintenance work within the lungs, so that more damage to lung tissue can take place, due to cigarette smoke, for example. No amount of alcohol is safe.

Despite what has been repeated for many years, drinking alcohol does not prevent heart disease. *The British Journal of Medicine* analyzed the scientific data collected over many years, and found that even one drink a day not only did not protect against heart disorders, but it contributed to them. Generally, people choose alcohol in order to relax and feel better. The program given in this book can help you do just that, without the increase in risk that taking alcohol gives.

Alcohol, then, really is a poison, in any amount. Drink some, and have a biopsy taken from your liver, and under the microscope, you will see death to some liver cells. Your liver is trying to keep this poison out of your bloodstream. The liver is enormously regenerative; you can cut two-thirds of it out, and the whole thing will regrow in six weeks. But why make it do that, in the name of relaxation? Should we have

23 miserable hours per day and one "Happy Hour" a day, caused by poisoning ourselves? What is wonderful about the program in this book is that by simple breathing exercises, you can feel better immediately, without drinking poison in order to do it.

Alcohol suppresses vital functions of your immune system. Therefore, its use is particularly associated with increased risk for cancer: cancers of the lungs, mouth, esophagus, stomach, breast, prostate, and liver, especially when taken in conjunction with cigarettes. No amount of alcohol is safe. Even one glass a wine per day increases risk for breast cancer. If you use the techniques given in this book, along with following the dietary suggestions, you may be able to protect yourself or recover from lung diseases along with so many other disorders, avoiding the potentially dangerous side effects of alcohol.

CAFFEINE

Drinking caffeine can make your lung problems worse. In the short run, it does dilate bronchi, and can help during an asthma attack. However, as it wears off, it can then make you more susceptible to episodes. It increases adrenaline, temporarily, but as it wears off, beginning at four hours, you end up feeling MORE TIRED. Caffeine can also make you feel more nervous, something that having a lung disease itself may induce. Caffeine makes you feel worse, and even if you have a temporary uplift, you may ultimately feel more depressed. Like sugar, caffeine is a very socially accepted form of a highly addictive "upper" drug. Caffeine is a stimulant chemical. It makes the central nervous system more active, so you feel more awake. However, it also makes you feel jittery. It actually decreases blood supply to your brain. Because it stimulates the release of dopamine in your brain, you feel temporarily happier; but once it wears off, you feel more depressed. You can elevate your mood more effectively by doing the breathing exercise program given in this book, which will increase your dopamine levels in a more sustained fashion.

Our national coffeehouse fascination may be contributing to the obesity and diabetes epidemics in the world. Caffeine increases insulin secretion making your blood sugar go up above normal, and then drop down below optimum, leaving you first energized and then depressed. It raises your blood cortisol, which makes your body store fat, especially around your belly. At first, you may not feel as hungry, but its use is associated with weight gain, partly from the increases in cortisol, but also because you become more hungry when it wears off. Elevated cortisol levels interfere with your immune system functioning. Therefore coffee intake has been associated with increased risk for cancers of the lung, breast, prostate, bladder, kidney, and pancreas. Coffee may also predispose to the formation of digestive irritation and ulcers. Black tea and coffee increase the risk for fibrocystic disease of the breast, which in turn may elevate your risk for cancer of the breast three to fivefold, and also make it more likely you would need a breast biopsy at some point in your life to analyze these lumps for cancer.

Decaffeinated coffee or tea drinks also contain significant amounts of caffeine; a cup of regular coffee or black tea has about 80 mg of caffeine; decaf may have up to 30 mg. Drinking caffeine is hard on digestion: it acts initially as a laxative, but when it wears off, it can cause constipation and irritation of the rectum. Although green tea contains less caffeine than black tea or coffee, it still has about 30 to 50 mg per cup.

Coffee and regular black or green tea have been promoted as sources of anti-oxidants, the elements in our diets that help prevent aging, but there are better sources in drink choices without caffeine. The high temperatures used to roast the beans has been found to increase cancer-causing chemicals called acrylamides, prompting the state of California to consider a warning label for coffee cups. The anti-cancer element found in green tea, catechin, may better be taken from other sources, such as fresh fruits, to avoid the caffeine still present even in the decaf version. Chocolate is naturally bitter, so even the 70 percent form has 30 percent sugar added. Even if sweetened with stevia, chocolate contains about 6 mg of caffeine, and may interfere with sleep, as well as leave you more depressed. Carob powder is naturally sweet, higher in protein, and once you get used to it, can give you chocolate-like satisfaction without side effects.

In addition to the detrimental effects of sugar, they contain caffeine and many soft drinks have as much as 50 mg of caffeine, and are associated with obesity (especially belly fat) and increased risk for cancer of the pancreas, as well. Aspartame, found in sugar-free diet sodas, has an even higher risk of obesity and belly linked to its ingestion, along with an increased risk of depression, due to aspartame lowering levels of

Superdrink Smoothie

By adding certain nutritionally dense foods to the basic good vegan diet, you may enhance your intake of nutrients to assure your health. You can take Superdrinks, made in a blender, once or more daily, especially if you are having any difficulty eating an optimum diet.

You will need a blender. In it, place the following SMOOTHIE ingredients:

1 to 2 bananas as a base (frozen if you prefer thicker consistency)

1 cup ice cubes

½ cup fresh dark greens, such as kale and spinach

(Other vegetables, such as beets, parsley, watercress, carrots, celery, green peppers, can be used)

½ cup sprouts

1 tablespoon oat bran

1 tablespoon carob powder for chocolate-like taste (Optional)

1 tablespoon plant-based protein powder*

1 teaspoon nutritional yeast flakes *

1 teaspoon lecithin powder*

1 teaspoon fresh flaxseeds

1 teaspoon powdered multi-vitamin formula*

½ teaspoon bee pollen*

½ teaspoon bee propolis (produced by bees, it boosts immunity)*

¼ teaspoon fresh ginger and/or garlic

¼ teaspoon turmeric powder

Blend together to desired consistency, and enjoy. Serves: 1 to 2

Variation

Along with the bananas, add any of your other favorite fruits as desired

*Available in most fine health food stores.

serotonin (our hormone of tranquility). "Diet sodas" should be labeled "Weight-gain Sodas!"

Here are some foods and drugs which contain caffeine: coffee (even decaf), black tea, green tea, white tea, oolong tea, Red Bull and other "energy drinks, chocolate, Excedrin and other headache remedies, and PMS remedies.

CHOOSING WHOLE FOODS

So what *is* best to eat and drink to help you prevent and treat lung problems? The answer is relatively simple, though it may not be easy for you at first. The way the food occurs in nature is the way to eat it. The body does not need animal protein or fats; a diet based on these foods does not confer any advantages and does not make us stronger. You can find the testimonials of vegan athletes on the internet, who have shown better function after the switch of diet.

Choose the foods you eat each day from the new, best "four food groups": *One serving equals one-half cup.*

- Whole fresh fruit: 3 to 4 servings daily

- Whole fresh vegetables: 3 to 5 servings daily

- Whole, fresh-cooked grains: 1 to 3 servings daily

- Legumes: (beans, green beans, lentils, green peas, soy products such as tofu or tempeh), 1 to 3 servings daily

Add plenty of fresh herbs and spices to your meals. Ginger, curry, turmeric, oregano, garlic, onions, cloves, fennel, cinnamon, cayenne all have been found to boost immunity, and help with lung function.

YOUR DAILY MENUS

These whole foods can be combined in a variety of ways to create daily menus that are not only healthy, but also tasty. Here is a template of choices:

- **Breakfast:** Fresh whole fruit, whole-grain cereal without any added sugar (such as fresh oatmeal or rolled oats lightly toasted in a toaster oven); bean burrito, scrambled tofu; or vegetable and bean soup—actually a great breakfast, especially in the winter; tempeh vegan bacon

■ **Lunch:** Raw vegetable salad and sprouts with a dressing of lemon and garlic; soup, such as pea, bean, lentil or vegetable with tofu; whole grain pasta; sweet potatoes

■ **Dinner:** 3 to 4 steamed fresh vegetables, whole grains or whole grain pasta entrée with added beans, lentils, peas, tofu or tempeh

■ **Snacks:** Any fresh whole fruits or vegetables—for example, cherry tomatoes, sugar snap or snow peas, carrots; small amounts of raw nuts and seeds; popcorn with curry, garlic, basil or other herbal

Nutritional Summary

Here is a summary of the best dietary changes you can make to help your lung function, as well as your overall health. When planning your meals, remember to avoid meat, poultry, fish, eggs, dairy, sugar, alcohol, caffeine and decaf and instead choose these substitutes:

● **Avoid Animal Foods.** Meats, chicken, fish, dairy products, eggs; instead have clean sources of protein, such as beans, peas, green beans, lentils, dal, soy products, and raw nuts and seeds. Eggs and fish do not contain fiber, and may contribute to the growth of unhealthy bacteria in your gut as a result.

● **Avoid Foods Containing Trans Fats.** Don't buy anything that has hydrogenated or partially hydrogenated fats on the label. Use only very small amounts of cold-processed virgin olive oil in your foods.

● **Avoid Fried Foods.** When oils are heated to high temperatures, they can become toxic to the liver and other organs and interfere with immune system action. Steam or bake instead.

● **Instead of Refined Sugar.** Avoid all added sugars, including corn syrup, agave, fructose, maple syrup, and honey. Instead, use fresh fruits to sweeten foods, and small amounts of stevia as needed in drinks; chewing gum flavored with stevia can be a portable quick dessert seasoning; frozen whole fresh fruits, hot herb tea, herbal water with fresh lemon, lime, or cucumber; iced herb tea; herb tea placed in freezer, then blended into sorbet

■ **Liquids:** Your most optimum liquid to drink is water. Making sure you get at least the basic eight glasses a day of straight plain fresh spring water, which is best. If you want a flavored liquid, make it in addition to this stable amount. Choose herbal teas which have anti-inflammatory, immune-enhancing, and anti-cancer activity; for example, a turmeric tea "latte" made from the spice turmeric, with added black pepper for better absorption, and unsweetened almond milk instead of dairy, is a great morning pick-me-up for which your lungs will thank you!

substitute—mint flavors wake you up and can satisfy your "sweet tooth" without putting your teeth at risk from the side effects on the gums of eating refined sugars.

● **Instead of Alcohol.** Choose sparkling water and add fresh lemon or lime.

● **Instead of Coffee and Chocolate.** If you like the flavor of coffee, you can use a grain-based coffee substitute, such as the brands Roast-aroma, Pero, or Tecchino; they come as tea bags, as well as forms that you can put in your capsule-based or loose grind coffee maker. Chocolate contains caffeine, so it can interfere with sleep and leave you more depressed: unsweetened carob powder has more protein, and is a better choice.

● **Instead of Black or Green Tea.** You can choose any herbal tea, and avoid the detrimental effects of caffeine or even decaf. Turmeric, black pepper, ginger, mustard seeds, cinnamon, cloves, cayenne, cumin, fennel, and lavender can be used by themselves or in combination, and they act to boost immunity and make your phlegm thinner. Chamomile both reduces anxiety and acts as an antidepressant: it's a liquid glass of cheer! It's not just for insomnia, which it helps alleviate, but it can help whenever you feel stressed; you can make it extra strong, using three teabags, if you are having a particularly challenging day.

SUPPLEMENTS AND HERBS
TO HELP WITH LUNG FUNCTION

You can obtain most of your nutrition from a plant-based, whole foods diet. Since lung disorders can be an extra challenge to your body, the following supplements and herbs may be helpful in providing support to your immune system, circulation, and overall well-being.

Taking a daily multiple vitamin-mineral supplement has been debated for years, with the recommendations going back and forth. As of the latest scientific data, a complete multivitamin daily has really been shown to add years to your life and life to your years. With the science behind us, let's look at the specific vitamins and herbs your body needs on a daily basis.

Vitamin and Mineral Supplements

Vitamins are defined as small quantities of certain elements of the diet found to be essential to health. Fifteen vitamins have been determined to be required; eight are called "essential," since the human body can't produce them on its own and needs to ingest them in food. Minerals, such as iron and calcium, have also been found to be necessary components of your diet. Here are the vitamin and minerals most helpful to lung health:

Vitamin B. B vitamins are used up whenever you are challenged by stress, such as experiencing a lung problem. You can take one 50 mg multi-B before breakfast and another before lunch and you may find, as do so many of Dr. McLanahan's patients, that you have more energy almost immediately. Avoid taking beta carotene as a separate supplement, since some research has linked it to an increased risk of lung cancer.

Especially if you choose to be vegan, take 1,000 mcg of vitamin B_{12} daily. B_{12} is found in soil, but our food has become so clean we do not always get enough in the diet. The sublingual form is most well absorbed, and is especially recommended for those over age 50, who may have a harder time absorbing B_{12} from the gut.

Vitamin C. The body uses vitamin C to help with tissue repair and fighting infections. Add 1,000 mg of vitamin C complex, and increase up to your bowel tolerance (it will cause diarrhea), then back down to a stable intake, usually around 3,000 to 5,000 mg per day. Research has shown that taking extra vitamin C not only helps prevent respiratory infections such as colds, but also shortens their duration.

Vitamin D. Vitamin D_3 is the active form of vitamin D. Most Americans are low in vitamin D_3. If you live above the latitude of Georgia, even if you get a lot of sun exposure in the summer, (your body can make vitamin D when your skin is exposed to the sun), you will run low of levels in the winter. Take about 1,000 IU daily, and have your blood levels tested to see if you might need more.

Herbs

Your lungs can benefit from taking herbs in your diet, including basil, oregano, rosemary, and turmeric. You can also take them in the form of herbal teas, which boost your immunity, as discussed on page 51. In addition, you can take herbs in supplement form to boost immunity and assist in lung health. Start with very small amounts, as people vary with their amount of sensitivity. Cinnamon, for example, may provoke allergic reactions. Rarely, lavender also affects certain persons.

Garlic. Eating fresh raw garlic gives you the most benefit for your lungs; start with very small slivers, and increase gradually to 1 to 3 cloves daily. (You can use parsley or xylitol flavored chewing gum to mask the odor in your breath.) If you can't tolerate garlic in this form, you can eat it cooked; but if neither of these works for you, capsules of garlic oil or deodorized garlic, 1 to 2 capsules before meals, will help you prevent infection and increase your immunity. The most effective form contains allicin.

Nettles. The herb stinging nettles has been found to be a great remedy for allergies and asthma. It acts by stabilizing your immune system's mast cells, which produce histamine. Taking nettles acts therefore as a natural antihistamine, without any side effects. Begin with 500 mg of the dried or freeze dried whole herb, twice daily, and increase as needed. Dr. McLanahan has had many patients who have experienced relief from allergic congestion, and even seen their asthma disappear, by using this natural approach. Scientific research has documented this herb's effectiveness.

FASTING AND YOUR LUNGS

Fasting is a way to assist your body in its maintenance and repair work. Whenever you eat, a significant shift in blood supply goes down to the digestive tract, to attend to the processes of digestion. Relatively less is given to the brain, making you feel sleepy after a meal. For this reason, many spiritual traditions have recommended fasting as a means of staying more mindful and awake during religious days, and for making more progress in meditation.

The old adage, "Starve a fever, feed a cold," is the result of a distortion by history. The original proverb was: "If you feed a cold, then you'll have to starve the fever." So the initial message back then was that it is best to fast for both conditions. The advisory proverb about fasting and illness has been changed to a half-truth.

Fasting, either when you have a cold or a fever or no matter what your illness makes physiological sense. Since viruses, bacteria, fungi and other bugs harmful to us are more vulnerable to food deprivation than your body's cells, fasting helps your body get rid of them. In addition, if the body does not have to send blood to digestion, these resources can be focused on fighting the infection. It's as if, when you stop taking guests in through the "front door," (your mouth), your body is able to send its resources to clean "closets"(your tissues)—to do whatever repair work your body needs to achieve good health.

Use hot water with lemon and cayenne, ginger tea, or garlicky tomato soup. Do not drink any sweet fruit juices; diluted orange, grapefruit, or lemon juices are acceptable.

Scientific studies have shown that fasting lowers levels of circulating insulin, helping to prevent metabolic syndrome and diabetes type 2. Fasting also lowers levels of Insulin-like Growth Factor 1 (IGF-1), a blood element of which high levels are associated with aging and cancer. Animals that fasted regularly live longer and develop less chronic disease.

Fasting has also been shown to increase blood levels of Brain Derived Neurotropic Factor (BDNF), low levels of which are found in Alzheimer's. This factor acts like an antidepressant: Fasting makes you feel good! Fasting has been documented to lower blood pressure and elevate mood. In one study, fasting even one day per month decreased risk for heart attack by 42 percent.

The liver stores enough protein for two weeks; do not fast for more than that, or your body will break down your own muscles to get protein. Do not fast without first checking with your doctor, and never fast without drinking plenty of water, at least eight cups per day.

CONCLUSION

You can commence to eat more mindfully right away, and begin to reap the benefits on your breathing. Although individual variations can be present, these are the general guidelines that have been found to be more important. Try one food at a time, to see if it makes your symptoms better or worse. If you can't comfortably fast for a full day, try eating earlier at night to allow more time for an overnight fast period. Yes, we are what we eat, and also what we digest and circulate optimally! You don't have to eat cardboard-tasting foods for the rest of your life to remain healthy. More and more, tasty whole food options are now available. Take a deep breath, choose well, and enjoy!

Chapter 4

Lifestyle & Adjunctive Treatments to Improve Breathing

In this chapter, we will look at other lifestyle modifications and natural actions you can consider using to help you take deep breaths. Whether called "'integrative," "functional," "complimentary," or "adjunctive medicine," these additions to the conventional interventions of drugs and surgery have scientific support and are available in many medical centers. Most medical schools now have departments of integrative healthcare, and research is abundant to support their use. Here are the elements we consider your best options.

OVERALL STRESS REDUCTION AND YOUR LUNGS

Everyone needs to address their stress levels, but particularly to prevent and treat lung disorders. Both acute and chronic stress can affect the health of your lungs. For one thing, whenever you feel stressed, you tend to breathe faster and in a more shallow manner, which can leave you not only feeling more short of breath if you already have lung disease. As your breathing becomes less deep, the total air exchange becomes less effective—which can also bring on asthma attacks. For another, it can also affect the ability of your immune system to fight infections—one of the reasons why students get more colds at exam time.

The breathing exercises in this book can lower your stress levels, and teach you how to keep your breathing slow and deep even when you are challenged by stressful situations.

Stress can contribute to as much as ninety percent of illness. It can impair the balanced functioning of your body and mind directly, or it can lead you to make unwise decisions in your lifestyle. The breathing exercises presented in this book can directly address your stress levels. Even one set of the exercises changes the body and mind, makes you feel better, and helps you breathe better too. Start with a daily breathing practice, and as you will see in this chapter, there are some other natural approaches to help you keep your stress levels to a minimum:

PHYSICAL ACTIVITIES

The right type of physical movement has been shown to reduce stress. The problem always seems to be how to find the time to make it part of your daily or weekly routine. Once you start any of the following suggested activities, you may be able to experience a sense of relaxation and a lessening of stress.

Exercise. Exercise itself reduces stress, see Part Two. If you have difficulty walking or breathing well at rest, within your capacity, you can do some active aerobic exercises and weight training just in a chair. When possible, take an elevator to a floor above and walk down, go to a gym and work with a trainer, bike, swim, dance, play a sport, join a class, and use the internet to find ideas. All of these actions have been shown to help lower stress levels.

Get and Give Massages. Both giving and getting massages has been documented to reduce stress, and increase endorphins, our natural painkillers. Endorphins are hormones produced in the brain, nervous system, and gut that link to our natural opiate receptors to create a feeling of pain relief and well-being.

Add Extra Deep Breathing and Alternate Nostril Breathing. Take a moment to breathe deeply whenever you are feeling stressed, and do extra breathing practice throughout your day, as presented in Part Two.

Do Extra Deep Relaxation. Add extra sessions of the mind-body relaxation technique of Deep Relaxation, see page 165. Follow the guidelines given there to add this practice into your daily life, where you check out the tight parts of your body, stretch, tighten and release them, and feel the benefits.

Do Stretches. Start simply, have a yoga teacher come to your home or attend a class for gentle or beginner yoga; aim for a little stretching every hour.

MENTAL ACTIVITIES

Just as there is a physical course of action you can take to lessen your stress, there are also mental techniques you can use to reduce your tension. Many of these approaches have been used for centuries throughout the world to find inner peace. Others are more contemporary in their approach, but can work just as well.

Meditate. A quick 10-minute meditation can help reduce physical and mental tension. With the body and mind relaxed, the immune system circulates better. Meditation can benefit your lungs in the following ways.

The practice of meditation can help you relax, and when you do, the capacity of your lungs to do repair work is increased. When you are stressed, your blood supply is shunted more to your muscles, brain, and heart, and less to repair work. Regular meditation can help you breathe more easily all day long.

"Meditation" is defined as the act of concentrating and quieting the mind. We are all "meditating" all the time. We think about 300 to 1,000 thoughts a minute. Our constant chattering mind often contains stressful thoughts about ourselves, others, events, the past, and the future. The formal practice of meditation aims to bring our awareness to our habits of thought; slow down and relax; analyze and replace any negative cycles of thinking with more encouraging ways of looking at things to help us improve, especially in the content of lung health, our state of relaxation, and our daily lifestyle choices.

See page 159 for instructions in meditation, and aim for at least two sessions a day. Take it easy, make it fun, and eventually incorporate a meditative aspect to everything you do: walking, using your phone, and singing in the shower.

Physiological Effects of Meditation

Every thought we think has a physiological effect. As we improve in being able to quiet and direct our thought stream, the health effects of mediation can be measured. Even a few minutes of practice lowers respiratory rate, heart rate, and blood pressure, as you become more relaxed. Your muscles release their tension and inflammation is decreased, as can be measured by C-Reactive Protein levels in the blood. The stress hormones adrenaline and cortisol are lowered, while the relaxation hormones endorphins, serotonin, melatonin, oxytocin, and dopamine are elevated. Activity in the right and left brain becomes more balanced, and the EEG is more synchronized, both of which are associated with a more relaxed physiology. Increased alpha, theta, and gamma waves can be measured on EEG recordings.

Even areas of your brain are changed in size by regular meditation: the prefrontal cortex, where good decision-making is centered, and the hippo-campus, associated with memory become larger. The amygdala, larger when you are under more stress, becomes smaller. The speed at which your brain can function, measured via IQ testing, becomes faster, and the amount of cortical thickness that usually declines with age and is associated with your ability to think well, actually increases in volume. The ends of your chro-mosomes, called "telomeres" become thicker, helping protect you from cancer. The expression of 500 genes has been found to be affected. This new area of understanding, termed "epigenetics" means that you are not stuck with the diseases associated with your genetic inheritance. Whether or not you express these genes, they can be affected by your lifestyle.

Practice Visualization. See yourself healthy, and doing what you love. We visualize all the time, whenever we think of a picture in our mind's eye. The formal practice consists of consciously choosing to image a healing light or happy place within, to help you relax. See page 159 for more details.

Pray. For many people, even a short prayer can replace worry. Connection to your spiritual beliefs can make you feel less alone and see your problems within a larger and more reassuring perspective. Scientific research has demonstrated the benefits of prayer, both when asking for support and praying for others.

Change Your Attitude. The way you see yourself and the people around can either put a smile or a frown on your face. By finding practical ways of uplifting your spirit, you can minimize your negative feelings and replace it with a more positive attitude. It takes work, but it's well worth the effort in reducing stress.

See the Good. How might the stressful event be beneficial? When you look for the silver linings playbook in everything, you can become less tense, and this can help in your healing process. The body is so connected to the mind that every thought you think has a physical effect. Positive thinking is not just wishful thinking, but shifts your physiology to assist your path to wellness.

Look for Signs. What positive messages can you find? Again, looking on the bright side can not only encourage you to stick to a healthy lifestyle, but change the functioning of your body. Circulation, blood pressure, immune function, and more are impacted by the thoughts you hold.

Live in the Moment. Easy to say, but it actually reduces stress significantly. Let go of thinking about the past or future. Notice the "now." Feel the benefits of the Golden Present. Depression can come from focusing on the past and anxiety from dwelling on the future. If you shift your mind to present moment awareness, you don't have to carry theses stressful habits. You don't have to hope for a better future, you can find things to be grateful for right now.

Live as if You Already Have What You Want. This relaxes you. This is a fast way to shift your habits of mind. Because your body reflects your every thought, and you think between 300 to 600 thoughts per minute, having your mind anticipating a future event creates the stress of worrying whether or not it will come about. By picturing a successful outcome, athletes and businessmen have learned that it helps them stay relaxed during the process of fully achieving the goal. Basketball players, for example, that visualize their free throws going in the basket have a higher shwoosh rate. Your body reflects whatever you hold in your mind, so if the pictures are positive, you can stay relaxed while you are on your healing journey.

Learn to Say No. In a kind way, say "I'd love to, but I can't." Often, the pressure to have others' approval can lead to the stress of taking on more work or choosing unhealthy options in lifestyle. This sentence assures the other person or persons that we appreciate them, but honors your own needs to live a balanced life and maintain your healthy choices.

Pretend. Even faking it can help reduce stress levels. This means that even when you don't feel like laughing, you can pretend to smile and laugh to cheer yourself up. One study showed that persons who were asking to make themselves laugh three times a day for five minutes lowered their stress levels. You can use this principle to help with anything you want to accomplish; act as if it already is achieved, and you will relax more and be able to more easily move towards you goal.

PRACTICAL ACTIVITIES

Have you ever noticed how you feel when someone has told you a funny joke? For that moment, the laughter you experience sets you free of the stress you may have been carrying around all day long. As it turns out there are a number of everyday things you can do to experience that same feeling. Here are a few things you can do reduce the stress.

List Your Goals. Write down five things you want to do and detail the baby steps to get them done. Sometimes even daily goals can seem beyond overwhelming, especially when you are ill. Organizing them into smaller steps, which you can more easily achieve, can give you a genuine sense of accomplishment, and can help you stay relaxed in the midst of action. You can keep updating this list as you go along; it helps you become more clear about your daily practices and other important lifestyle considerations.

Write and Draw. Keep a journal, art book, or coloring book. All have been found to reduce stress. Again, when you can become more exacting about your aims, and document your ups and downs, the greater sense of control you have helps you stay positive in the midst of it all. Imagery, such as coloring uplifting pictures or sayings, has been shown to lower blood pressure and boost immunity.

Keep a Gratitude Journal. Write as many things you are grateful for as you can, and update it at the end of each day. Being grateful has been shown to activate a different part of the brain than that which is associated with worry. Focusing on the positive things in your life helps motivate you to take the difficult steps towards ongoing consistent healthy lifestyle choices.

Have a List of Relatives or Friends to Call. Choose more than a few. We are social creatures. Lack of feeling connection and experiencing loneliness is the number one emotional stressor associated with disease, as outlined in Dr. Dean Ornish's inspiring and important books *Love and Survival* and *Undo It.*

What is one of the worst things we do to those in prison? Solitary confinement is extremely difficult. When we have others cheering us on, it becomes easier to stick with the necessary lifestyle actions for health. You can look for a support group at your local religious institution, Whole Foods or health food store, health club, or online. Even just finding one lifestyle buddy can help make a difference in your success. Aim to find one trying to be healthy or with whom you feel genuinely supported and encouraged.

Give Without Any Expectation of Reward. Be a Secret Santa daily; it will make you feel much better, increase your joy of life, and decrease your sensation of stress.

Sing. Whistle while you work works! Singing activates the brain differently, and gets you out of the worrying habit. Called "Music Mind," singing, chanting, or whistling uplifting tunes shifts the activity of the brain. It shifts from worrying, centered mainly in the left brain, to a relative activation of the right brain also, which does not experience time and space in the same way, but simply lives more in the present moment.

A therapy group has even explored having participants sing their problems into a microphone, making up a song that begins with lines such as, "Oh, I'm having a hard time with my husband," making it easier to laugh at places in your life in which you may be stuck. In addition to reducing your stress, it can be a pleasant way of exercising your lungs. Actively playing music or singing is most effective, but just listening to music you find comforting and inspiring can help; music therapy has been scientifically demonstrated to have many health benefits, and can even improve surgical outcomes.

Add Laugher to Your Day. Live on the funny side, the funny side of life. Laughing often, especially at yourself, reduces your stress immediately. And while this may sound strange, even fake laughter works. You can try placing a pen cross-ways in your mouth to make you smile. After just a few seconds, you may notice you start to feel better. Smiling activates higher levels of endorphins and serotonin, our feel-good hormones. So does laughter.

In one study, subjects who were requested to make themselves laugh five minutes three times daily had lower depression and anxiety scores, lower blood pressure, and even lower cholesterol. Not only does laughter change our physical functioning and hormone levels, but can exercise our lungs and just make us feel better. (See the inset Laughter and Your Lungs on page 65.)

Get a Pet or a Stuffed Animal. Anything that makes you laugh. Those who own pets have fewer asthma attacks, probably from how much joy and relaxation they obtain, which offsets allergic exposure. You can choose a hypoallergenic breed. If you can't have an actual animal, a toy that you can actively pet can be soothing, or you can watch pet videos on YouTube or the phone or computer app Reddit, which has abundant funny, beautiful, and inspiring animal clips.

Do Something Healthy and Fun. Be silly, choose a healthy kind of fun, like getting a slinky or yo-yo. When you think of yourself as youthful, and do things that make you laugh, your body begins to shift. In one study, where seniors spend a weekend dressed in poodle skirts and other clothing of their youth, and danced and acted as their joyful younger selves, measures of their blood pressure, memory, and stress levels were all improved just in a few days. Also, when you are doing any activity you love, such as dancing, you can exercise your lungs without as much physical and psychological effort.

While you don't have to do every one of the suggested activities we've mentioned, you can try doing one or two. You will be the best judge as to how they work. As you perform any of these activities, don't be afraid to switch around. You should discover quickly which ones work best for you. Those should be your keepers, but always maintain an open mind for other activities that provide you a sense of joy, the very thing that diminishes tension.

Laughter and Your Lungs

Laughing can be a kind of nutrient in its own right. Have a five-minute hearty laugh break, taking a longer class or internet session, choosing comedies, or whatever makes you laugh regularly can help you take a deep breath! It can be an important and joyful addition to a healthy lifestyle that helps to prevent and treat lung disorders. You may not feel at all like laughing, but once you get started, even fake laughter can act very quickly to help you feel better. (It's hard to sustain fake laughing for very long before you are really chuckling and then guffawing at yourself.)

Laughing uses the same muscles as exercise; strengthens your core and lower back muscles. Laughing can get you breathing more deeply, strengthening your respiratory muscles; helping prepare you for the breathing exercises program given in this book, and bring a quick form of stress management into your life.

Laughter lowers your blood pressure; the blood pressure goes up for about 30 seconds, then it becomes lower. Your respiratory and heart rate also are elevated slightly for a short time, then reduced. Laughing increases your protective hormones: serotonin, the hormone of tranquility; endorphins, our natural painkillers; and dopamine, associated with a feeling of bliss. The immune system elements interleukin and NK cell activity have been documented to increase. The hormones associated with stress, adrenaline and cortisol, are lowered after a session of laughing. The blood's level of the amount of inflammation in your body, C-Reactive Protein, is lowered. Elevated blood sugar is decreased, and the carbon dioxide levels in your lungs are diminished.

Your mood is marked enhanced; both anxiety and depression are diminished. Even a fake smile was found to lower stress hormones. In one study, even fake laughter, performed three times a day for five minutes, lowered cholesterol, blood pressure, and helped relieve anxiety and depression. When you smile, the muscles in your face don't have to work as hard: it takes 18 muscles to smile and 37 to frown. If you laugh regularly, your risk for heart attacks and irregular heartbeats (arrhythmias) is forty per cent lower! Even anticipating a funny event lowers stress hormones for three days ahead of time.

PREVENTION OF RESPIRATORY INFECTIONS

Any infection adds distress to the lungs' accomplishing their functions, especially if you already have a lung disorder. You need to take actions to prevent and treat the effects of harmful viruses, bacteria, and fungi. Fortunately, a number of simple measures can help you avoid infection, and some adjunct remedies can help if you do develop a disease.

Hand-washing Helps. Do extra hand-washing. If you are in public, cough or sneeze into a tissue or your elbow crease rather than your hands, to avoid spreading any germs. Avoid those who are sick, and stay at least six feet away from anyone who is sick. Because of how common influenza has become, mainly if you have a lung disorder, call a doctor if you develop respiratory symptoms, especially if you run a temperature. Check with your doctor to see if a flu vaccine makes sense for you. Flu continues to be contagious for about one week.

Eat the Right Foods. Eat lots of fruits and veggies, and do your best to avoid refined sugars, white flour, and white rice. Even one tablespoon of sugar (anything except stevia) causes your white cells to be less active. This lasts for hours after you eat that cookie or cake—choose fresh fruit as your sweet treat instead. Also avoid fruit juices and dried fruit, since they likewise affect blood sugar, and increase risk for diabetes and gum disease. Whenever the blood sugar is above normal, you are more vulnerable to infection. (See pages 44 and 45 for details.)

Avoid Caffeine, Alcohol, and Other Drugs. Caffeine temporarily boosts your feeling of energy by a drug effect, but ends up leaving you more tired and vulnerable. Do the breathing exercises given in Part Two of this book instead.

Fast One Day a Week. Fasting has been shown to boost immunity by diverting your energy from digestion to repair work. It also reduces risk of heart attack and cancer by as much as 50 percent. Depending on how active you need to be, fast on water with cayenne and lemon (2 tablespoons of lemon juice and 1/10 tablespoon of cayenne pepper; no maple syrup or other sweetener), diluted fresh fruit or vegetable juice, or whole fresh fruits or soup. See more about the benefits of fasting, on page 54.

Get Enough Sleep. Less than 7 hours per night has been shown to lower immunity. See the section on massages to get a good night's sleep, on page 33.

Stay Warm. Colds and flu are more common in winter for three principle reasons: First, the viruses which cause them are more easily killed by the heat of summer. Second, exposure to a higher number of germs takes place in winter's close quarters and less-ventilated rooms. Thirdly, research has shown that getting chilly, especially if your feet feel cold, does increase risk for catching a cold or flu. Warm hats, gloves, and scarves can help, but the most important thing is warm and dry socks and boots.

Take a Steam or Sauna at Least Once a Week. Not only does this increase circulation of your disease-fighting white cells, but also increases their numbers and potency. Even a sauna or steam once a month has been found to decrease risk for heart disease and cancer by as much as 50 percent. Just stay in only as long as you are completely comfortable; a few minutes to begin with.

Enjoy Garlic Breath. Chewing 1 to 2 cloves of raw, fresh garlic per day boosts immunity. Take it in very small bits to begin with, until you become used to it. If raw garlic is too much for you, try the cooked or baked variety, or take the capsules or deodorized capsules, 1 to 3 per day. See further discussion on garlic, page 53.

Use Aromatherapy. Lavender aromatherapy helps you relax and boost immunity. You can combine four drops each of lavender, eucalyptus, and bergamot essential oils in an 8-ounce glass spray bottle. Fill the remainder of the bottle with water and shake well. Spritz the air around you 4 to 5 times every couple of hours. These essential oils kill bacteria, viruses, and yeasts.

Take Vitamin C Complex with Rose Hips, Vitamin D, and Zinc. Recent research has shown that vitamin C does prevent colds; take 1.000 mg 2 to 3 times daily. Vitamin D_3 also helps the immune system fight infection; start with 1,000 IU daily. Zinc, 50 mg daily, boosts immune function.

Use a Neti Pot. Since most colds and flu bugs enter through the nose's mucous membranes, the "neti" pot helps wash away such viruses and bacteria, before they have a chance to make you ill. Health food stores carry these special tools, shaped like a teapot, or you can simply use a small teapot. Fill with warm distilled water, add a pinch of salt, tilt your head to the side and slowly pour the water into one nostril. It will reach the back of your nose, and then come out through the other nostril; repeat on both sides. Breathe through your mouth while you do it; you can feel quite refreshed and breathe more easily and openly afterwards.

Increase Your Time in Breathing Practices, and the Chest-Opening Stretches. Follow the guidelines given in Part Two of this book. The breathing exercises strengthen your lungs to resist infection, and the stretches stimulate the thymus, a gland at the base of the throat that helps with the growth of T-cells, one type of your immune system's fighter white cells.

Move Your Body. Keeping your body physically active, exercising to the point where you sweat, at least 30 minutes daily, helps the circulation of white cells—your body's immune elements that patrol your body via the bloodstream and destroy harmful germs before they are established. Try fast walking, dancing, running, biking, swimming, or other sports you enjoy. Do not overexert, however, because that can lower immune resistance.

Have Fun. Make plans for fun. Even looking forward to something fun has been shown to boost immunity for three days ahead of time. If you can, avoid stressful situations; if you can't get out of them, develop an inner bubble of calm to deal with such challenges. Stress weakens immunity, while happiness strengthens it.

Laugh. It's no joke. Laughter really does increase immunity, white cells become more numerous and more active; antibodies to fight infection are increased. Even fake laughter helps. See more on laughter, page 65.

Do Service. Altruists boost their immunity, and helping others boosts the immunity of those you help as well. Both giving and receiving a massage (once you have washed your hands) activates the immune system, so schedule time for both.

Stay Optimistic. An optimistic attitude activates immunity: music, colors, and art that uplifts you changes your physiology in a positive direction, makes you feel better and increases the number and activity of your white cells. Give yourself a happy self-talk, and have happy talks with others.

NATURAL TREATMENTS FOR RESPIRATORY INFECTIONS

Any infection needs to be checked out by a healthcare provider; especially if you already have a lung disorder. However, you can use the following home remedies to assist in your healing. They have been scientifically shown to work, and can support the use of conventional approaches, to overall help you feel better and get well faster.

Stop Working. If you feel yourself developing a sore throat, runny nose, fever, or muscle aches and pains, stop working and attend to your health until these symptoms are gone. First, you may be spreading whatever you have to the others working in your area. Second, using up extra energy to work simply depletes those important nutrients necessary to fight the infection.

Take Plenty of Fluids. Fluids will help your immune system circulate white cells, and make up for any fluid loss associated with fever. Plain water or herb teas are best; coffee and black or green teas are dehydrating. Aim for 8 to 10 8-ounce glasses of water daily or more if you feel thirsty.

Gargle With Salt Water. Do this every 10 to 15 minutes, until the throat stops being sore. Salt disrupts the membranes of invading bacteria, viruses, and yeasts, while not harming healthy tissue. Use organic sea salt for best effect.

Chew a Fresh Garlic Clove. This helps immediately eliminate the pain of a sore throat, due to the sulfur content of the fumes, which serve as a natural antibiotic, and the overall immune boost of garlic.

Eat Lemons and Chew Lemon Peel. In addition to the vitamin C, another substance in lemon, termed "limonene," especially found in the peel, has potent anti-viral, anti-bacterial, and anti-fungal activity. Make certain the lemon is organic.

Sweat. If your temperature goes up, check with your doctor— fevers need to be reported. Make yourself sweat by increasing room temperature and crawling under a bunch of comforters. Germs that give us disease live comfortably at 98.6, the body's normal temperature. A fever, as we now know, is the body's effort to create conditions that make these bugs more vulnerable to your immune system removing them, as well as speed up blood supply so that more white cells can attack.

Fast Until You Begin to Feel Better. Not eating makes physiological sense, since viruses, bacteria, and fungi are more vulnerable to food deprivation than the body's cells, and if your body does not have to send blood to digestion, it can focus its resources on fighting the infection. Never restrict fluids; drink plenty, especially hot water with lemon and cayenne, ginger tea, or garlicky tomato soup. Do not drink any sweet fruit juices, since they elevate blood sugar too much; diluted citrus juices can be helpful. Do not fast for more than a day or two unless you check with your doctor.

Do a Localized Steam Treatment. Take a pot of water, put a lid on it, and boil. Take it off the burner, place a towel over your head and the pot, take the lid off, and inhale the steam for 20 minutes. You can add some drops of eucalyptus, lavender, or tea tree essential oil, which directly kill offending germs. These sessions can greatly reduce a cough, and help you sleep better at night.

Take Honey for Cough. A teaspoon of honey not only helps the medicine go down, as Mary Poppins sang, but it is the medicine. Studies have shown that it works better to stop coughing than commercial preparations. Never give honey to an infant, and limit your intake to a few tablespoons per day, as needed for cough.

Take Extra Vitamin C, Vitamin D, and Zinc. Increase your Vitamin C complex with rose hips to 2,000 mg three times a day (take less if you get diarrhea); this has been shown to cut the amount of time of a cold in half. Take 4,000 IU of vitamin D, and 50 mg of zinc, three times daily until you are better.

Take Herbs. Echinacea does work. Hundreds of scientific studies have documented its ability to increase numbers and activity of white cells, and decrease the time of illness. Take two droppers or three capsules of the dried herb, four times daily. Astragalus is an herb also shown to boost immunity; take two droppers or capsules twice daily.

Do not try any home remedy without checking with your healthcare provider first. However, these are simple and care actions you can take that can help you on your way to full health. Take it easy, and don't overdo it or strain yourself. Try one action at a time, and monitor your body's response. These simple yet powerful approaches can help you prepare for the breathing and meditative practices given in this book.

ADJUNCTIVE TREATMENTS

Beyond the lifestyle changes we have discussed, a number of other drug-free treatments have shown themselves to be effective in treating many breathing disorders. If improving your breathing capacity is a priority, it is important to know what all your options are.

Acupuncture. The science of the practice of acupuncture began in China about 2,000 years ago. One of the reasons it has lasted has been its remarkable success to relieve pain and quickly help patients recover. Scientific study now supports its use for a variety of illnesses. It may be able to help you breathe more easily, and make you more able to take deep breaths. Small needles are placed at specific points around the body, and sessions usually last from one-half hour to one hour. Don't worry, the needles are generally very small, and the slight sting of their insertion quickly passes. Sometimes, electrical current may be attached to the needles for increased benefit. Sessions can be as frequent as three times a week in the beginning, transitioning to once a month, for maintenance, later. Results may differ with each practitioner, so you may have to try more than one. Acupuncture has been scientifically documented to help with asthma and COPD.

Aromatherapy and Taking a Deep Breath. The nerves in your nose that allow you to distinguish fragrances are directly connected to the area of the brain where stress and emotional memories are principally stored. Therefore, smells can carry associations from your childhood and be utilized to help you relax. For example, the fragrances of vanilla and lavender have been scientifically shown to assist in evoking relaxation in most people. These and other essential oils can be added to your massage oils, placed in a misting plug-in atomizer or sprinkled onto your pillow at night. (Since they are water-based, they do not stain). The scents of fruits—grapefruit, lemon, lime— and mints—peppermint, spearmint, wintergreen—help you feel more awake. You can drink peppermint tea when you want to feel energized and lavender-chamomile when you need to unwind. Jasmine and Ylang Ylang are others that assist relaxation. Vanilla scent was demonstrated to help patients relax during the stress of X-ray and MRI tests.

You can try from the array of essential oils to see which ones help you feel most comfortable. Some people are allergic to specific fragrances, although this is rare. Just to be safe, therefore, be certain to try them in small amounts at first.

Chiropractic and Osteopathic Adjustments. Adjustments made by a chiropractor or osteopath can really help your breathing: they can assist you in taking a deeper breath because you are more relaxed. They are overwhelmingly safe, with complications being extremely rare. Tension is relieved in your muscles and spine usually via a soft thrusting motion, although some practitioners achieve corrections in posture and balance using simple pressure or small devices, and avoid such movements altogether. Especially if you have neck or back pain, these modalities have been scientifically documented to help provide relief.

Nasal Dilator Strips. Something as simple as strips that are attached to each nostril, to pull them more open, can help you take a deeper breath by enlarging your nasal passages. These can be applied whenever you feel short of breath, have congestion or swollen nasal passages, or can be routinely used as prevention, especially at night. These strips have been scientifically studied, and both subjective and objective improvement documented. One brand, the "Breathe Right" strips are widely available at local drug stores and online. You may notice you sleep better and wake up more refreshed with their use.

Oxygen Tanks. Oxygen tanks can deliver more oxygen than is found in normal air. The amount of oxygen can be up to 100 percent, and given via prongs that fit underneath the nose, or most efficiently, with a mask. This supplemental oxygen can be used as needed, but it may serve as a relaxing placebo for a mild disease, and thus can be psychologically rather than physically addictive. The best way to use oxygen tanks is to monitor your breathing, and followed by your healthcare provider with regular blood tests. Types of machines are available that convert ambient air to increase its oxygen content, dispensing with the need for actual tanks filled with oxygen. The sizes of these machines have decreased greatly, making them smaller than a backpack and easily portable.

Hyperbaric Oxygen Treatments. In a specialized chamber or via a face mask, oxygen can be delivered at a higher pressure. Retired football quarterback Joe Namath, now 76, credits his ongoing recovery from the memory brain effects of his many concussions to having over 140 sessions of hyperbaric therapy. Research has not yet established efficacy of such treatments for COPD and other lung disorders, but some anecdotal evidence suggests it may have benefit, though the effects may also simply be psychological, as a placebo. Some side effect risks have been found, though they are generally minor and short-lived. Eyesight changes include acceleration of existing cataracts, and hearing loss, temporary or ongoing, may occur. Major problems, such as lung rupture and seizures have rarely developed. Therefore, further research is needed to see if delivering the oxygen via mask may offset these complications of therapy.

CONCLUSION

Scientific research now supports the effects of lifestyle choices on your lung function. An American College of Lifestyle Medicine has been founded to further education and research in these areas, and most medical schools and centers now provide integrative medicine services. What we recommend is beginning with diet: move towards a plant-based diet as soon as you can, and away from foods found to be inflammatory, especially dairy, meats, and eggs. Add supplements that have been documented to help lung function, such as nettles, and choose to get a massage when you can. You will be able to more easily take deep breaths all day long, so that you can improve your quality of life most effectively.

Chapter 5

Why Breathing Exercises Work

& Avoiding the Excuses for Doing Them

When our bodies are called upon to move quickly, we naturally deepen our breaths. This acts to strengthen the diaphragm and the other muscles that help with our breathing. We all need to exercise daily to achieve optimum health and healing. In addition, the program of breathing exercises given in this book helps in a unique and different way. It improves not only the health of your respiratory system, but your overall health as well, via mechanisms that are different from simple active exercise and strength training. Relaxation itself is healing, and these exercises help you feel more relaxed right away.

In this chapter, the science behind the breathing practices is given. In order for you to take a deep breath most easily, it does help to actively include varying types of exercise into your daily life. However, the *Take a Deep Breath Program* especially can give you and your respiratory system an extra edge, and help you create the very best health from the inside out.

AEROBIC TRAINING

The fact is, too many of us lead overwhelmingly inactive lifestyles—sitting at work, sitting in cars, and sitting on couches. However, by including some daily periods of active aerobic exercise, it has been shown that these type of exercises have profound effects on health. The word aerobic means "in the presence of oxygen," and refers to exercise that improves circulation of oxygen into your tissues. In addition, while twenty minutes is the least with which you can get by, it doesn't have to be all at once. Simply walking fifteen or twenty minutes to start off makes a difference. If you can't walk distances, you can try taking the elevator to the fifth floor of a building, and then walking down to the ground level at your own pace, or going to a pool and walking in the water for a few laps. If you are a little more mobile, you might try a comfortable stationary bike, moving to music while in a chair, or even just bouncing your legs using a mini trampoline while you sit in a chair next to it.

The goal is to get your heart rate up. Like any other muscle, the heart gets stronger with exercise. The muscles that help you breathe also get stronger, and it will become easier for you to take a deep breath. Don't strain, just keep the pace where you can talk comfortably. Using music along with your exercise has been shown to help you exercise longer as has having one or more buddies to keep you company help keep you at it. If you can afford it, have one session or more with a personal trainer. Remember how important it is: you can expect to add quantity and quality to your life, about 3.4 years of additional life expectancy, in better health, for simply exercising 20 minutes daily.

HIGH-INTENSITY INTERVAL TRAINING (HIIT)

When you are ready for something a bit more strenuous, consider high intensity interval training. It has been found to be the most effective type of aerobic training. It's the way animals and children exercise: bursts of action, followed by relaxation. It keeps things playful: think of skipping along as a kid. Whatever action you are doing, go as fast as is comfortable for a 1 to 2 minutes, followed by 5 minutes of slow, easy pace. You can feel more conditioned and fit most readily by adding this method into your exercise plan.

Here are the steps for HIIT:

• Stay comfortable, proceed only at your own pace

• Speed up your exercising for 1 to 2 minutes

- Then go back to a slow pace for 4 to 5 minutes

- Repeat this alternating of pace for 10 to 20 minutes, while mindful to stay comfortable and avoid overexertion

STRENGTH TRAINING

Strength training focuses on making muscles stronger by pushing or pulling them against resistance. You can do this using machines, stretch bands, or simply by doing sit-ups and push-ups; at least three times a week can really make a difference in your overall health. Not just do your muscles get stronger, but also your metabolism becomes more efficient. This can help in the overall maintenance of your respiratory system. Scientific research has demonstrated the benefits of regular strength training for persons suffering from COPD. To get motivated to practice, you can seek help from a personal trainer, or find tutorials on YouTube and other places online. (See Resource section on page 173.)

THE SCIENCE BEHIND THE BREATHING EXERCISES

While these methods of exercise are essential, the rewards of the breathing exercises given in this book are unique and work in a brilliantly different way. Their regular practice can help prevent and heal not only lung problems, but they affect the health of the entire body. Plus, they just make you feel so much better that the effort to practice them becomes something to which you look forward. You don't have to wait; you can feel better *immediately*. Now, take as deep a breath as you comfortably can. Notice that you feel an increased sense of relaxation right away. There is a scientific explanation behind this feeling, as we shall see.

These breathing exercises work differently from the movement-based exercises we have just reviewed. Instead of increasing tension, they relieve it. They don't require as much action. Their movements are simple and without strain. You end up feeling more refreshed, rejuvenated, and relaxed. The physiology of these exercises is in contrast to the forms of active exercise: they help you renew yourself from within, and instead of feeling tired after a "work-out," you feel energized from a "work-in."

SIMPLE DEEP BREATHING

What exactly is happening when you just take a deep breath? In quick summary:

- Your respiratory muscles are strengthened

- You activate a response called the Hering-Breuer Reflex

- The increased state of relaxation from this reflex affects your entire body

- Your stress hormone levels go down

- It becomes easier to take another deep breath

Respiratory Muscles. Let's begin with the respiratory muscles. Like all muscles, they become stronger with use. For example, when a cast is put on an arm, and left there for six weeks or so, when it is taken off, the arms muscles are much smaller, shrunken from disuse. When an athlete wants to "bulk up," lots of reps on machines that require muscular activity are included. Whenever you simply take a deep breath, you are making the muscles of your respiratory system larger and stronger. The programs in this book are specifically designed to gradually make this activity easier and more effective.

Hering-Breuer Reflex. The Hering-Breuer Reflex is activated every time you take a deep breath. Stretch receptors, located in your lungs, are triggered by the expansion of your chest. They then fire a signal to our brain, which in turn acts to increase the activity of your vagus nerve, the largest nerve in the parasympathetic nervous system.

Increased State of Relaxation. Once the action of the vagus nerve is increased, a wide array of organs are affected in the direction of relaxation. You feel more relaxed right away. Your body also has more of a capacity for self-healing, since your blood supply is shifted: when you are stressed, the body diverts its energies to be ready for Fight or Flight response, sympathetic nervous system engagement. Blood is diverted from digestion and the liver, from the basic maintenance functions of the body and its immune system. That's one of the reasons people get more colds and other infectious diseases when they are stressed. Your nervous system and hormones shift towards the immediate defenses of running away or directly confronting a stressor, rather than fighting off invader viruses or other bugs.

Stress Hormone Levels Go Down. So you can help to prevent and treat infections, auto-immune, and other disorders simply by doing the deep breathing presented in this book. The hormone adrenaline is increased whenever you experience short-term, alarming immediate stress. Adrenaline acts to make you feel more tense, a way of being ready for action against the stressor. It increases your breathing rate, making your respiration more difficult.

Long-term stress can increase cortisol levels, leading to further diminish immune activity, and causing your body to pack fat in your belly because it wants to be ready for periods of famine, should they develop. Unfortunately, this inflammatory fat in your belly does not just affect your appearance, but increases your risk for depression, diabetes, heart disease, cancer, and Alzheimer's. Fortunately, simply doing the deep breathing given in this book can lower your cortisol levels, and help you reverse this trend.

Taking Another Breath Becomes Easier. Because you feel more relaxed from even one deep breath, it becomes easier to take another. In addition, as you learn to stay more relaxed all day from your daily practice, it becomes more possible to make the other healthy choices, such as other types of exercise and dietary wisdom, required to optimally maintain your health.

One patient was having a very hard time in their life, and a friend helped him both laugh and begin a path of healing. The friend said to remember the phrase, "Dude, just take a deep breath," whenever things were challenging. You can apply that to both genders.

BELLOWS BREATHING EXERCISES

When you rapidly contract your abdominal muscles, forcing the air out of your body, and then passively allow the air back in, this breathing exercise helps you wake up, and improves circulation in the respiratory system and your whole body. It's a great way to start the day, or do whenever you need to feel more energized.

This type of breathing exercise increases the activity of the sympathetic nervous system, though not in the way stressful events would. Because just your breathing is involved, your body can circulate its oxygen where it is needed for repair: when you are doing aerobics or strength training it will simply go to the muscles involved, and some to the heart and respiratory system. When you are doing the bellows breathing, more oxygen can be given to the digestive organs, liver, and immune activity because your body is overall staying relaxed.

Your metabolism is increased, making this type of breathing recommended especially for those struggling with being overweight. Instead of that extra caffeine break, you can try a bellows breathing session with better long-term effects on your fatigue levels.

ALTERNATE NOSTRIL BREATHING

In this exercise, presented later in Part Two, you use your fingers to alternative closing off first one nostril, and then the other, while keeping your mouth closed. It may at first seem weird to alternate which nostril your breath comes through. For inspiration, you can refer to the YouTube on which Giselle Bunchen, supermodel wife of Super Bowl winning quarterback Tom Brady, demonstrates how to do this type of breathing on the Jimmy Fallon late night talk show. The science behind its benefits has been firmly established, and you can make it a fun daily practice. (See Resource section, page 173.)

This type of breathing exercise is balancing and calming, and can be done daily to help you experience and maintain these feelings. Breathing through the right nostril increases activity of the sympathetic nervous system, while when you breathe through the left nostril, it activates the parasympathetic system. Alternating between the two helps you balance their function, and leaves you feeling awake and yet relaxed, calm and yet ready for action.

Doing this practice at least twice a day will prepare you to take on and then let go of the inevitable ups and downs you face. Especially when you are in need of releasing your stress, you can take a few minutes and transform anxiety or depression into a sense of the joy possible in any moment, find the silver linings playbook within it all.

Now that you have some knowledge of why breathing exercises work, you may still find yourself making excuses. Sound familiar?

OVERCOMING RESISTANCE TO PRACTICE

When we commit to practicing the gentle stretching movements and breathing exercises regularly, we discover the cumulative effect they have on the body and mind. Not only does our breathing improve, but we find we have greater peace of mind and better coping strategies for times when we are short of breath. You may ask yourself, why don't I do the exercises every day? Well, we are human! We make excuses for ourselves even when we know the benefit of the exercises. Sometimes, we may simply feel tired and unmotivated because of our illness. I don't have to tell you that being short of breath is debilitating and can cause depression as well. Be gentle with yourself, but don't give up on regular practice.

The following section discusses various common excuses people use to avoid being regular in the breathing practices, and offers some tricks to help you transcend them.

I Don't Have Enough Time

This is the most common complaint of all—because it's true! Twenty-first century culture is crazy busy. The next time you are feeling overwhelmed and pressured for time, remind yourself that you still can, and should, squeeze in some exercise. Do a little pursed lip breathing or a short meditation, which you'll learn more about later. If you choose to do some physical movements, remember that you don't have to do every exercise or sequence every session in order to make your routine count. It's much better to do a simple, short practice every day than it is to do a long, intense practice once or twice a month. You also may find you prefer certain exercises more than others. That's fine. All that means is that your intuition is helping you discover what you need.

Making time to practice regularly can actually make time seem to expand! By improving your physical and mental capabilities and awareness, solutions to problems will become more obvious, and the length of time it takes you to perform various activities will be reduced. In short, you will feel like you have more time.

I Don't Have a Place to Do It

I challenge you to make one! You probably have a special area with a desk where you pay your bills. Likewise, you have a place in the kitchen or the dining room (or in front of the TV) where you take your evening meal? And of course, we all love our beds. These are special areas in the home that are dedicated to specific patterns in our daily life. Practicing your breathing exercises in a similarly dedicated space can inspire us and make us more regular.

While most of the exercises in Part Two can be done anywhere, anytime, you may find it easier to remember to do the practice when you've dedicated a small area for it. All you really need is a chair, a mat, a block, and a strap. Beyond that, you may enjoy lighting a candle and offering a prayer or an affirmation for healing. If you like to have music playing, be sure it's not too exciting or distracting. My favorite meditative music these days comes from an ensemble called "A Winged Victory for the Sullen." More suggestions can be found in the Resource section.

It's Too Noisy in My Home and Neighborhood

Noise can be a distraction when you're trying to focus on your practice. It may help to get up a little earlier than your family, or your neighbors, or before the milk delivery trucks start rumbling through the streets. We've all heard the axiom, "Accept the things you cannot change, change the things you can, and have the wisdom to know the difference." Taking these words to heart can help you analyze the quietest time of day, informing you of the best time for your routine. And use a little quiet music in the background if that helps to keep your focus on your practice and not on the hustle and bustle of the awakening world.

My Kids (or Grandkids) Interrupt Me

This can be a good thing! It's an opportunity for you to engage them in your wellness routine. Let them know that you'll have more energy to play with them if you do your routine every day. Encourage them to join you and ask them how it feels, and tell them a little bit about how you feel when you practice. If they get bored doing the routine with you, keep a basket full of quiet toys or crayons and paper for them so that they can stay close to you (which is what they want) but not cause a disturbance.

I'M TOO STIFF FOR EXERCISE

If shortness of breath has taken a toll on your body's natural strength and flexibility, you may feel intimidated to try the exercises. Have faith in the "righting reflex," the natural capacity of the body to correct and heal itself. The gentle stretches we have designed for you will naturally strengthen your muscles, rid your body of toxins, and accelerate your body's natural healing capacity.

You have to start somewhere! If you're stiff, so be it. Learning to accept and love your body as it is right now is also essential.

Discomfort from Overeating

Have you ever noticed how your shortness of breath is exacerbated after a heavy meal, laden with carbohydrates? It's because as the carbohydrates break down into sugars and are metabolized, they form excess CO_2. This sends a signal to increase the rate of breathing to deal with balancing the gases. Having this knowledge can help you make better food choices. It may help to weigh and measure your food intake—become a student of the affect food has on your COPD. These days, you can get very scientific data from apps on your phone or your fit bit that can illuminate hidden information about how your diet is exacerbating your shortness of breath. It's best to wait a few hours after a big meal to begin your practice.

I'm Scared I May Get Into a Jam!

One of the ways the breathing techniques can really help you is when you are out and about and you find yourself getting breathless from exertion. Because you're becoming a better observer of your body with your practices, you may notice you're getting in trouble before you start to panic. Panic turns on the stress hormones and creates a tightening in the lungs making breathing even more difficult. You can stop whatever you're doing that's causing the problem and start doing some pursed lip breathing. Talk to yourself as if you're a coach—"You know what to do here!" Having a regular practice of 20 minutes a day is key to establishing an automatic response to increased shortness of breath. And those 20 minutes can have a lasting effect for the rest of the day.

CONCLUSION

Much research—over a thousand scientific studies—has demonstrated the health and healing action of breathing exercises. You can modify them to suit your comfort level, but like any practice, the regularity can help you find the benefits. As Yogi Berra, champion baseball player and humorous sage said, "Ninety percent of success is half mental." Keep your breathing practices fun and steady, and you will reap the healthy rewards.

Now you have also learned some strategies to overcome the resistance to exercise—overcome the excuses we come up with— and the importance of these physical activities. In the next section, Part Two of the book, you begin your practice; the next chapter will spell out the equipment and appropriate clothing you will need to get started.

PART TWO

Physical Practices

Chapter 6

Beginning Your Practice

Now we're about to begin! You've learned so much about the lungs from the detailed information in Part One of this book, I know you want to see if these routines are really going to work for you, and hopefully they will. However, before you actually start the exercises, take a moment to look through this next section on props so you have what you need. It's a bummer to get all set to begin and then realize you don't have the proper shoes, or your pants are too tight. Have a look at this chapter so that doesn't happen to you!

COMMON PROPS

For almost every form of exercise, it's best to have the right equipment and appropriate clothing. For instance, I recently wanted to go for a hike in the woods near my home. After I put on my shoes, I realized my socks were too thin! It may seem insignificant, but I know how my feet appreciate good cushioning. So I had to take my shoes off, find a better pair of socks, and start over so that my hike would be a pleasure instead of a chore. The exercises in Part Two are no different—you'll want your props at hand. For our practices, we don't need a lot of the traditional exercise equipment. Most of what we are going to do can be done with things you have on hand. We don't want anything to get in the way of you starting to do breathing exercises. Here are a few things you might want to gather before you begin.

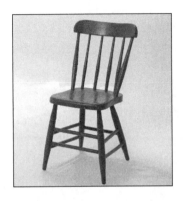

A Sturdy Chair

All of the stretching exercises and most of the strengthening exercises will be done seated in a chair. It needs to be sturdy, with a straight back. The seat may be cushioned for greater comfort. We will also be using the chair for the standing exercises, to avoid the risk of falling.

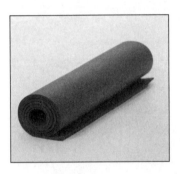

A Mat

Used under the chair, mats can be helpful to protect the feet and also keep the chair from sliding around. Now that Yoga is everywhere these days, Yoga "sticky" mats are readily available online, at sporting goods stores, and at the big box stores like Target and TJ Maxx.

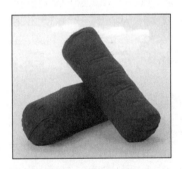

A Bolster or Pillow

During the chair routine, it's beneficial to have your feet on the floor. If you're a little short, place a block, or pillow under the feet for support. For the section on restor-

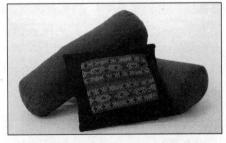

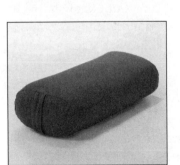

ative postures, you may want to invest in a larger bolster to give your body an opportunity to rest deeply in the restorative positions.

Blocks

Like Yoga mats, blocks used for Yoga can also be helpful, especially if you're unable to place your feet on the floor during the exercises.

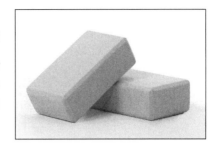

A Strap

When the body is stiff, a canvas strap can be used to "lasso" a foot or hand in order to gently bring the body into position. You can also use an old necktie which can be found at your local hand-me-down store.

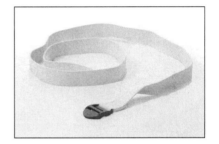

Comfortable Clothing

Sweatpants, Yoga pants, or pajama bottoms—what these all have in common is the stretchy waistband. Since we'll be bending and stretching, as well as expanding the belly on inhalations during the breathing practices, you'll be more comfy with loose fitting pants, a cotton T shirt, and a warm hoodie on top. You might want to keep a warm shawl handy for the guided relaxation, since we spend about 10 minutes resting and the body will naturally cool down.

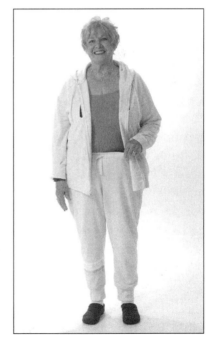

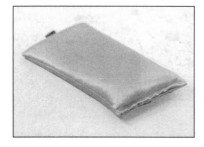

Eye Pillow

For the restorative positions and guided relaxation you may enjoy resting a soft eye pillow on your eyes. I especially love the ones made with a silk covering and the scent of lavender. Check in the Resource section for a retailer.

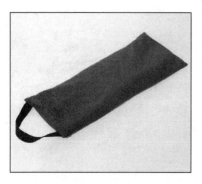

Sandbag

Not all of my students enjoy the feeling of heaviness when a sandbag is placed on the belly or on the feet in certain exercises, but I do! For me, it signals me to relax even more deeply. So I've included a sandbag in this group of things to have on hand. However, it's optional.

TIPS FOR GETTING THE MOST OUT OF YOUR PRACTICE

In addition to gathering and/or purchasing props and clothing, there are a number of things you can do to prepare for your breathing exercises, in order to get the most out of them. We all lead busy lives—getting to work, looking after our elderly parents, shopping, cooking, shuttling our kids to piano lessons—but these gentle practices can help put it all in perspective. The stress-relieving benefits of the exercises that follow will improve your COPD symptoms by improving circulation, increasing your endurance, and building energy levels so you can do more activities without becoming tired or short of breath. Here are some ways to maximize the benefits of your exercise sessions.

Practice on an Empty Stomach. Wait at least two to four hours after your last big meal and an hour or longer after a snack, before practicing the exercises. You want to assimilate all the benefits of your practice and not have energy drained away by the process of digestion. A meal heavy in carbohydrates increases carbon dioxide in the blood, making it more difficult to breathe. Rather than drinking water throughout your practice, wait until afterwards to enjoy a glass of water. This will help you shift your consciousness from a fully relaxed state to fully aware.

Shower. Come to your practice clean and empty. Try to have your morning elimination and shower before you begin. If you practice in the evening, have a change of clothes and a quick wash of your face and hands.

Remove Jewelry and Other Restrictive Items. If you wear a watch, large earrings, necklaces, and other jewelry, be sure to remove them so they don't get in the way. If you have long hair, keep a scrunchy or rubber band nearby to tie hair back if it becomes a distraction. Take off your belt, and make sure your waistband is sufficiently stretchy for maximum comfort.

Fresh Air. The room in which you practice should be warm and comfortable, but not stuffy. Open a window on a nice day to freshen the air. If you want to practice outside on a summer day, avoid doing so in direct sunlight in the heat of the day. Don't wear perfume, scented lotion, or anything else with a particularly fragrant scent—especially in public classes. Air fresheners, scented candles, and scented fabric softeners are made with harmful chemicals that are not helpful for your lungs, so ban them from your home! Therapeutic essential oils can be used in the privacy of your own home.

Alleviate Distractions. If you're at home, turn the phone on mute so you aren't listening for calls. Close the door so pets won't be wandering in. It helps to set aside a certain time every day as your "me time," and try to stick to a schedule. If you're practicing with others, keep your awareness within and don't try to compare your progress to anyone else's. You'll avoid injury and breathlessness by going at your own pace and paying attention to what you're feeling. Your ability to observe your body will be enhanced over time, and you'll find yourself bringing consciousness to every part of your body.

Shorten Your Practice if You're Pressured for Time. Keep yourself on a schedule that isn't too rigid. You don't have to do every movement in a sequence every day. If you only have time for a few exercises, at least do them rather than skipping your session altogether. At the very least, do 10 to 20 minutes of the breathing exercises every day. With practice, they become more natural and can have a lasting effect all day.

Gradually Build Your Practice. Initially, you may only be able to do a few repetitions of the exercises. It may take up to a year to increase your number of repetitions, so don't be discouraged if you don't see dramatic improvement right away. Lung disorders don't usually happen overnight, so be patient with yourself as you begin to improve lung function. Remember, the lungs have redundancy! The more you practice these routines, the more unused areas of the lungs will begin to wake up and function.

IMPORTANT CONSIDERATIONS

If you have other health issues, such as high blood pressure or arthritis, physical limitations because of your weight, or age-related stiffness, please check with your trusted medical professional before beginning these practices. Once you get the OK, you will want to take care not to overdo. My teacher had a phrase I love—"Take it easy, not lazy." You may start out like gangbusters, and then find yourself falling off the wagon. Don't be discouraged. Just start up again, and make a commitment to practice a little something every day. Soon, you'll regain that ease of movement and breath, feel stronger, and be mentally more alert. The ultimate benefit of this combination of movement and breathing is the peace of mind that is the natural result of mindful physical activity.

When we take time to exercise, our circulation improves and the heart gets stronger. As the cardiovascular system improves, endurance will increase and blood pressure will improve, bones get stronger, and sleep is deeper. Best of all, the gentle exercises we offer in the next chapter will give you more vitality and boost your self-esteem. You might even lose a few unwanted pounds! Don't you want to start right away?

Hopefully, you now have your chair, mat, block and other helpful goodies and are ready to start on the road to better breathing. The following exercise routines will be demonstrated by me, a regular person, not a super-model. If I can do these movements, you probably can do them too. Remember, you don't have to be young and thin. Let's do it!

Chapter 7

Exercises for Breathing Challenges

In this chapter, I will show you three different sequences of exercises to help you become more effective at taking a deep breath. These postures are so simple that even a beginner will be able to perform them! What's more, you can do these exercises anywhere you have a chair. Once you become familiar with them, you may find yourself practicing while you're at your desk when you need a little more vitality, by increasing the amount of revitalizing oxygen in your system. Building endurance using these gentle exercises decreases shortness of breath.

BASIC BREATHING TECHNIQUES

Aerobic exercise improves your heart function and strengthens muscles. Similarly, breathing exercises counteract tightness in the chest and allow the lungs to work more efficiently, allowing stale air to be released from the lungs and fresh oxygen to enter. Here are the basic breathing techniques that you will be using throughout your exercises.

Full three-part breath. Place your hand on your belly, below the belly button. Breathe into that area so that you feel your abdomen lift as you inhale. As you exhale, feel the abdomen collapse again. Next, you inhale into the low belly and then into the rib cage area. Exhale from the rib cage; empty the low belly as well. Now, inhale into belly, rib cage, and into the upper chest also. You may notice your collar bones lift slightly, but take care not to shrug the shoulders up toward the ears. In addition, when you breathe deeply, you also notice the side ribs expanding, and even the breath moving into the back of the body.

Pursed lip breathing. Using the same three-part breath we just learned, purse your lips and as you exhale, imagine you are exhaling through a straw. This helps to slow down the exhalation which increases the absorption of oxygen and breath. Over time, try to exhale about twice as long as the inhale.

NON-LOCOMOTOR EXERCISES

It's important to remember that the lungs are just one component of your breathing "factory." Also important is your diaphragm, a muscle that sits between your lungs and your abdominal viscera. It acts like a bellows, moving air in and out of the lungs. Your overall muscle tone is also important, and if you've stopped exercising because you really haven't felt up to it, don't worry, the exercises we're about to share with you are designed to be easy and doable. In this chapter, we will give options for strengthening muscles of the core, exercises to build flexibility in the joints, leg-strengthening routines to build balance, and—I know you're going to enjoy these—movements that will help train your body to relax and refresh. All of these exercises are non-lo-comotor—you don't have to get up and go anywhere.

When we stop exercising because of COPD, or any of the restrictive lung diseases, it affects all the systems of the body. The muscles get weaker which results in creating shortness of breath at lower levels of exertion. Inactivity is not the answer! The exercises we offer are gentle stretches that will increase flexibility as well as strength.

Be sure to speak to your doctor about these exercises and make sure you are on the same page. Ask for specific recommendations for exercise, and make sure you're taking all medications as they are rec-ommended by your physician. If necessary, use oxygen therapy during exercise to prevent shortness of breath or exercise induced hypoxemia, a condition in which the supply of oxygen is insufficient for normal life functions. You may have already experienced this, and it can be scary.

There's no need to put yourself in danger when you exercise, keep your breathing tube handy when you're in exercise mode.

The first segment will demonstrate exercises done seated in a chair. These are simple stretching exercises that will give you more flexibility in the joints while simultaneously building strength in the muscles that support the joints. This is important because when the muscles are weak, it places too much strain on the joints, leading to possible injury. (See available DVD in Resource section, page 173 for many of these same stretches.) Although on the DVD I demonstrate them on the floor, they are easily adapted for the chair.

The second group of routines will be done standing alongside a chair, using it for support as we bend, stretch, twist, and expand. These exercises will build strength overall, helping to create stability and vitality. Remember to stop if you start to feel short of breath, and resume when you've had a rest. But don't give up! If you have a good routine for doing these exercises regularly, you will build up to more repetitions. Plus, you'll start to feel a lot better!

Finally, we take some time in relaxation. Using props, which you'll learn about later, to get us comfortably into various positions, we will be guided into a dreamy state of ease and tranquility (See available website for free downloadable session in Resource section, page 173).

It's time to begin! Put on your comfy clothes, grab a chair and your yoga mat and follow me!

FLEX-ABILITY SERIES

This first series is ideal for anyone challenged with lung issues because it will help you increase the oxygen in your blood and build up strength without causing shortness of breath. Doing these exercises is important in building your awareness of how to breathe—remember, we normally only use $1/7^{th}$ of our breathing capacity in our everyday, normal breathing.

In the Flex-Ability sequence, stretches are done deliberately at a snail's pace, as if you were moving in slow motion. Each of the movements is dynamic—that is, coordinated with your inhalations and exhalations—and not static, or fixed. As a result, the sequence simultaneously tones the muscles that support your joints and helps rid your joints of toxins. The breathing component of the sequence also brings more oxygen and breath, the life force, into your body. Regular practice of the Flex-Ability series promotes a sense of lightness throughout your body.

The longer the exhale, the more benefit you gain, as the breath remains longer in the body. In addition to pursed lip breathing, another way to slow down the exhalation is to use the glottis in the hissing breath. This is a conscious partial closing of the glottis muscles at the back of the throat, just behind the larynx. The result is that the breath makes a soft hissing sound. The friction from the closing of the glottis creates heat in the body, which helps eliminate toxins. When used as a meditation tool, it calms the mind, and gives a good focal point for the restless thoughts. In addition, it brings good circulation to the throat, and is helpful in relieving sore throats. It is also said to improve the digestion and respiratory problems and bring a luster to the face.

SEATED SEQUENCE

The following nineteen exercises start with you sitting on a chair. Begin with your feet on the floor about twelve inches apart. Gently draw your shoulders up toward your ears, rotate them backward, and then release them. This will help open your chest and lift your sternum—the breast-bone. The hands can rest on the tops of the thighs.

As you perform the stretches, you should be conscious of your breath. Each inhalation should be through the nose, performed deeply into the abdomen. Your breaths should be full and noisy—that way, you won't forget to keep thinking about them! In contrast to most breathing, in the Flex-Ability series, you will be exhaling through your mouth using pursed lip breathing. This allows you to get a more complete exhalation. You can enhance the benefits of the sequence by imagining that every inhalation is bringing in fresh energy, and every exhalation is releasing toxins from your system. Included in the following exercises are routines that may relieve other physical issues from carpal tunnel syndrome to ankle mobility. Remember as you practice any of them, proper breathing practice will help you increase your oxygen flow.

- Flex and Point
- Book Feet
- Ankle Circles
- Knee Bends
- Hip Juicifier
- Shoulder Squeeze
- Love Your Fingers
- Wrist Wrangling
- Figure Eights
- Elbow Bends

- Thoracic Toning
- Side Stretch
- Side Twist
- Scarecrow
- Pelvic Tilt
- Chin Up, Chin Down
- Side to Side
- Ear to Shoulder
- The Finale

FLEX AND POINT

BENEFITS

Your feet form the foundation of your body—and it's important to keep your foundation strong! These stretches will help keep your ankles flexible.

TECHNIQUE

Inhale, and place heels on the floor. As you exhale, lift the heels and point the toes to the floor.

Repetitions: I recommend doing 3 to 5 repetitions of each exercise before moving on to the next. If you need to take a break before going on to the third or fourth repetition, go ahead and pause for a moment. Always be kind to yourself.

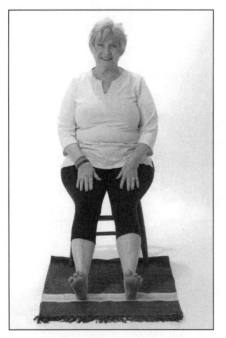
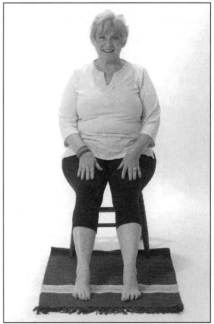

Start with heels on the floor   Lift heels and point toes down

BOOK FEET

BENEFITS

We don't often think of our ankles of moving sideways, but they do! By building lateral strength in your ankles you can help prevent injuries.

TECHNIQUE

Stretch the legs forward with the feet together. Inhale as you bring the soles of the feet close together, and exhale as you bring them wide again, imagine you are opening and closing the feet like a book.

Repetition: This is one repetition.

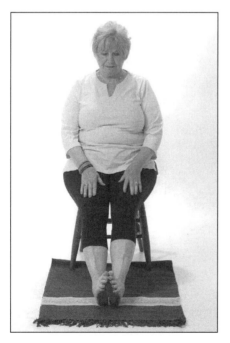
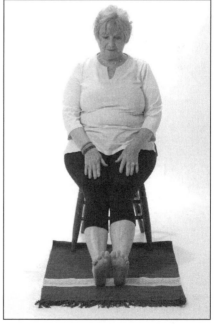

Bring soles together   Soles of the feet facing apart

ANKLE CIRCLES

BENEFITS

This exercise increases ankle mobility and improves circulation to the feet.

TECHNIQUE

With your feet side by side, draw circles with your toes, bending from your ankles. Inhale as you go downward, and exhale coming upward.

Repetitions: Do 3 to 5 repetitions in a clockwise direction, and do then do the same number of repetitions in a counterclockwise direction.

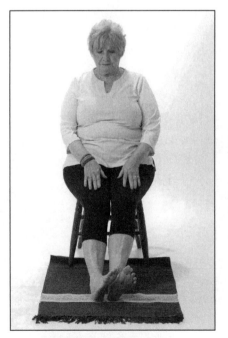
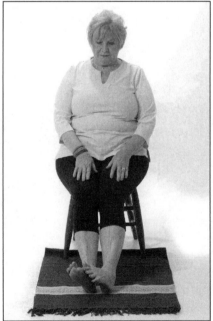

Feet side by side   Draw circles with toes

KNEE BENDS

BENEFITS

This exercise helps strengthen the muscles that support the knee. The gentle bending back and forth helps to restore flexibility to the knee joint, preventing injury.

TECHNIQUE

Begin with both feet on the floor. Inhale as you lift and extend the right leg, clasping the hands under the thigh. Exhale as you draw the foot back toward the chair.

Repetitions: Do 3 to 5 rounds and then switch to the other leg.

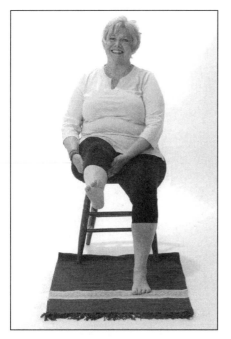
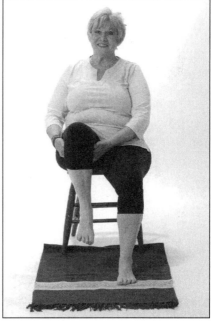

Lift and extend right leg   Draw foot back to chair

HIP JUICIFIER

BENEFITS

This exercise refreshes the synovial fluid within your hip joints, helping the bones glide effortlessly over each other. It tones the muscles of the leg, giving you a bounce in your step!

TECHNIQUE

Sit forward on the chair with the legs spread wide. Rotate the big toe of the right foot so it comes close or touches the floor. Sweep the leg to the left as far as comfortable. Inhale as you rotate the leg so the pinky toe touches the floor and sweep the leg back to the right. Exhale as you bring the legs close together, inhale as you go wide. Do 3 to 5 repetitions; then go to the other leg.

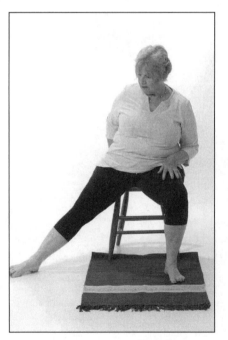 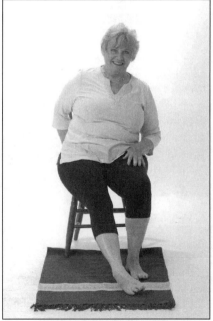

Right big toe touches floor   Left pinky toe touches floor

SHOULDER SQUEEZE

BENEFITS

This exercise tones the muscles around the shoulder joint, and also massages the area between the shoulder blades.

TECHNIQUE

Inhale as you bring straight arms up overhead, with the arms alongside the ears and palms facing each other; take care not to tense the shoulders up toward the ears. Exhale as you swing the arms down and behind the body, giving a little squeeze to the area between the shoulder blades. This is one round.

Repetition: Repeat up to 5 rounds.

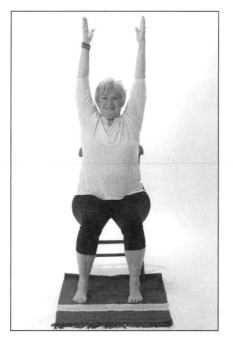 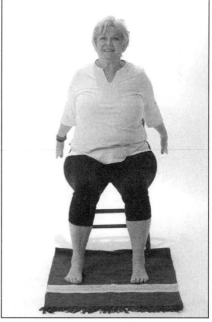

Arms straight up overhead   Swing arms down behind body

LOVE YOUR FINGERS

BENEFITS

This pose brings increased circulation to the fingers, helping to alleviate arthritis pain. In addition, it strengthens the muscles of the entire arm.

TECHNIQUE

Inhale as you bring your arms up level with your shoulders, fingers splayed and pointed upward. Exhale as you bend the wrists and squeeze the fingers into a fist. Take care not to tense up the shoulders.

Repetition: Do 3 to 5 rounds.

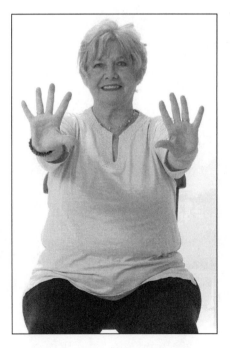

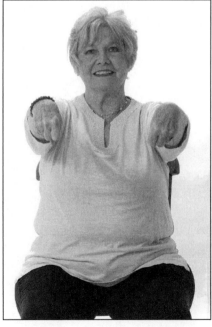

Arms up level with shoulders   Bend wrists, squeeze fingers into fist

WRIST WRANGLING

BENEFITS

This exercise helps to keep the wrists flexible and strong. It helps to make you a whiz at flying a frisbee.

TECHNIQUE

Keeping your arms tucked close to the body, bring your hands out in front of you, palms up. Inhale as you bring the sides of the pinkies close together, as if you were reading a book. Exhale as you rotate your hands at the wrist, so that the tips of the middle fingers are touching. Try to maintain the flatness of the palms and keep the elbows tucked in. This constitutes one round.

Repetition: Continue for up to 5 rounds.

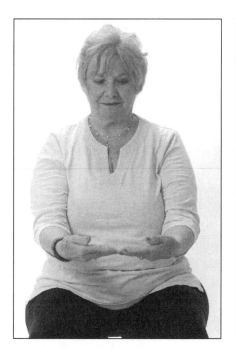
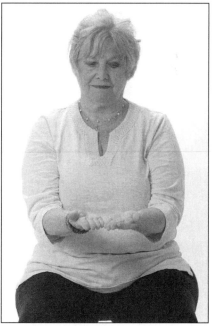

Hands out in front, palms out   Bring sides of pinkies close together

FIGURE EIGHTS

BENEFITS

This routine helps to prevent carpal tunnel syndrome and brings good circulation to the wrists.

TECHNIQUE

Make two gentle fists in front of you. While holding your fists together, begin making slow figure eights, inhaling as your fists move downward and exhaling as your fists move upward. Take care not to bring the elbows away from the body, rather keep them gently tucked to your sides.

Repetitions: Do 3 to 5 repetitions one way and then do the same number of repetitions tracing your figure eights in the opposite direction. It might be a little confusing to draw your eights backward, but you'll soon get the hang of it!

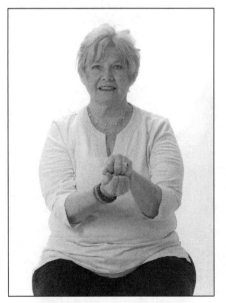
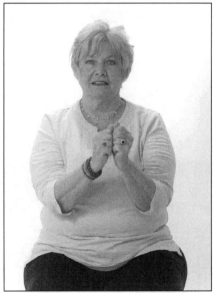

Make and hold fists together   Inhale, fists move downward;
exhale, fists move upward

ELBOW BENDS

BENEFITS

This exercise lubricates the elbow joints with synovial fluid, brings increased circulation to the joints, and strengthens all the muscles that support the elbow joints.

TECHNIQUE

Inhale as you extend the arms out with the palms up, about as high as the shoulders. Exhale as you bend the elbows and bring the fingertips to the tops of the shoulders. Keep the shoulder relaxed and down.

Repetitions: Do 3 to 5 repetitions.

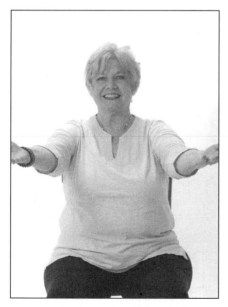 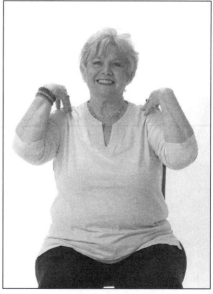

Extend arms out with palms up   Bend elbows, bring fingertips
                                        to tops of shoulders

THORACIC TONING

BENEFITS

This exercise is really great for keeping the upper back open and free, especially in the era of cell phones and computers when we are often hunched over, scrolling.

TECHNIQUE

Inhale as you touch the fingertips on the shoulder tops, bringing elbows close together in front of the chest. Feel the shoulder blades opening on the back side of the body. Exhale as you bring the elbows behind the body, squeezing the shoulder blades close together.

Repetitions: Try 3 to 5 repetitions

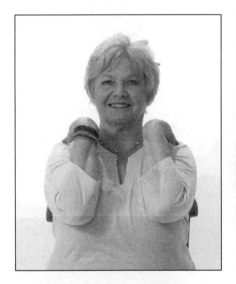
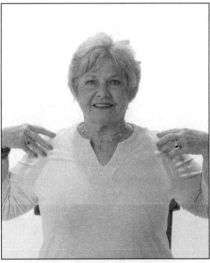

Bring elbows close together;   Bring elbows behind body;
touch shoulder tops   squeeze shoulder blades together

SIDE STRETCH

BENEFITS

This exercise gives a good stretch to one side of the body, while simultaneously giving a gentle massage to the other side. This helps to tone muscles that don't get used much as you sit at your desk all day.

TECHNIQUE

Inhale as you stretch your arms out to the side and lean the body to the left. Keep both arms soft and your shoulders low, palms facing down. Inhale as you bring yourself back to the neutral position. Exhale as you go down the other side. This is one repetition.

Repetitions: Try doing 3 to 5 repetitions

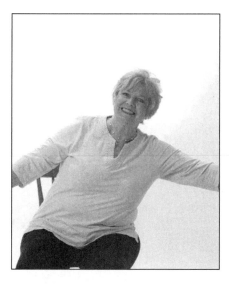 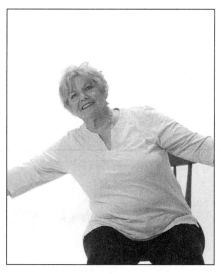

Stretch arms out, lean body to left   Stretch arms out, lean body to right

SIDE TWIST

BENEFITS

This exercise gives a good squeeze to the spinal column, helping to remove toxins and stiffness and bring fresh blood into the spine. The vertebrae in the spine are critical to moving and bending freely.

TECHNIQUE

Inhale with the arms out to the sides. Exhale and begin to twist the upper body to the side, bringing the head around last. Take care to keep the shoulders soft and not hunched up toward the ears. Inhale as you come back to the middle. Exhale as you twist in the opposite direction. This is one round.

Repetitions: Do 3 to 5 repetitions.

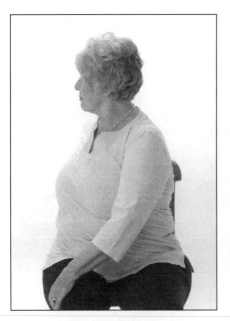

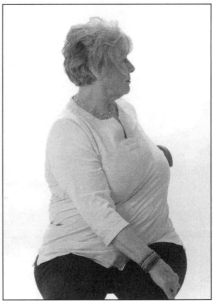

Twist upper body to one side   Twist upper body to opposite side

PELVIC TILT

BENEFITS

This exercise improves mobility in your lower and middle back. Arching the spine forward and backward increases flexibility and rids your joints of foreign substances that cause inflammation and may inhibit movement.

TECHNIQUE

With your feet on the floor and the legs wide, place the hands at the top of the thigh as you inhale and tilt the pelvis forward, squeezing the shoulders back and allowing the chest to puff out. As you exhale, move the hands to the knees and tilt the pelvis back, drop the chin to the chest creating a curve along the spine. This is one round.

Repetitions: This is one of my favorite moves, and I enjoy doing several repetitions, but only do as many as comfortable.

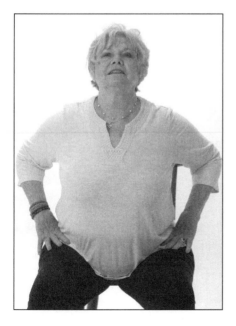 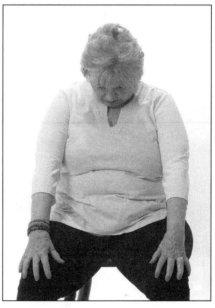

Head up, tilt pelvis forward   Drop chin, tilt pelvis back

SCARECROW

BENEFITS

The scarecrow exercise helps to strengthen and tone the muscles that support your shoulder area. By keeping these muscles strong, you increase you shoulder mobility and prevent rotator cuff injury.

TECHNIQUE

Inhale as you raise both arms up, as in "stick 'em up!" Forearms are perpendicular to the floor and the palms face forward. Exhale as you rotate your arms at the elbows and bring the palms parallel to the floor. Be careful not to let the shoulders tense and scrunch up by the ears.

Repetitions: Do 3 to 5 repetitions.

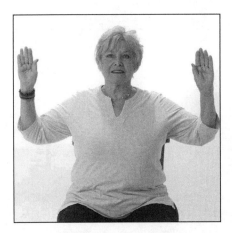   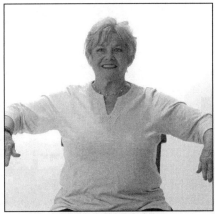

Raise both arms up,   Rotate arms at elbow,
palms face forward   palms face down

CHIN UP, CHIN DOWN

BENEFITS

So often when our neck gets a little stiff, we might rotate the head quickly, without much thought, as we try to release tension. In this exercise, we do the movements slowly and mindfully. This helps the muscles to relax more fully, allowing tension to dissipate.

TECHNIQUE

Inhale as you gently lift the chin about ¾ of the way up. You don't want to over-scrunch the back of the neck by bringing the chin too high. Exhale and slowly release the chin to the top of the chest.

Repetitions: Continue for 2 to 5 rounds.

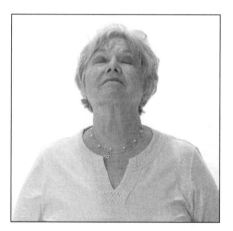 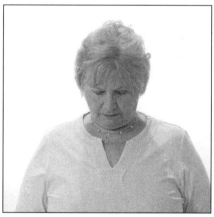

Lift chin 3/4 up   Release chin to top of chest

SIDE TO SIDE

BENEFITS

As with the previous exercise, Side to Side is done mindfully to bring good blood flow to the muscles of the neck. Don't go beyond your comfort zone, and have confidence that your flexibility will improve as you practice regularly.

TECHNIQUE

Begin with the head in neutral with the chin parallel to the floor. Inhale as you turn the head to the left to look over the left shoulder. Exhale as you return the head to the middle, then inhale as you turn the head to the right, looking over the right shoulder. Exhale as you bring the head back to the middle. This is one round.

Repetitions: Continue up to 5 rounds.

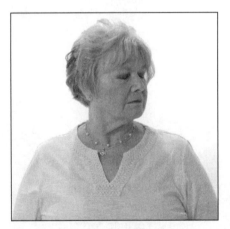
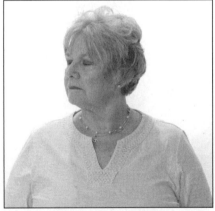

Turn head to left,   Turn head to right,
look over shoulder   look over shoulder

EAR TO SHOULDER

BENEFITS

This exercise brings a little squeeze to the sides of the neck, while simultaneously lengthening the opposite side, relieving muscle tension and increasing flexibility in all the vertebrae of the neck.

TECHNIQUE

Begin with the head in neutral, with the chin parallel to the floor. Inhale in this position. Exhale as you gently release the left ear down toward the left shoulder, facing forward throughout. Inhale as you bring the head back to neutral, and exhale as you drop the right ear to the right shoulder. Inhale back into neutral. This is one round.

Repetitions: Continue up to 5 rounds.

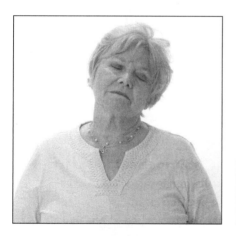

Drop head to left shoulder

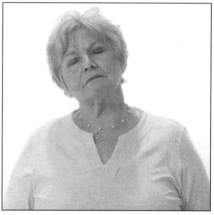

Drop head to right shoulder

THE FINALE

BENEFITS

You have completed all the flexibility exercises—Good for you! This last movement will signify that you have succeeded and will bring a flush of energy and joy into your chest. It will prepare you for standing up and getting on with your day.

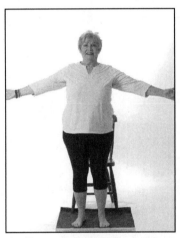

1. Extend arms out to sides

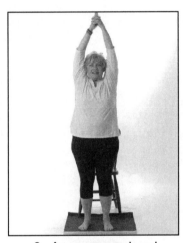

2. Arms up overhead

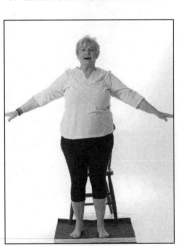

5. Extend arms out to side

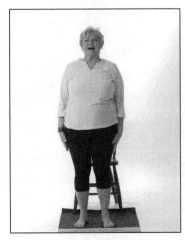

6. Lower arms down

TECHNIQUE

Inhale as you stretch your arms out to the sides and then up overhead. Hold the breath as you lock your thumbs and give a little twist to the right side, then to the left. Come back to neutral position and exhale fully and a little forcefully as you extend the arms out to the side again, lowering them down.

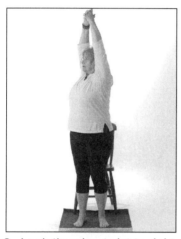
3. Lock thumbs, twist to right

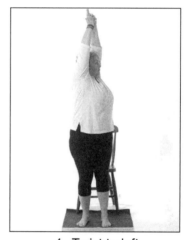
4. Twist to left

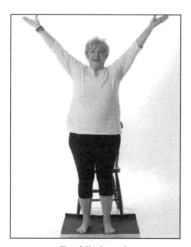
7. All done!

STANDING SEQUENCES

Next, we'll have a look at two routines in which we move the body from one shape into another, using the breath to initiate the movements. Based on a movement called the Salute to the Sun, the sequence can be done using a wall for support, or a chair. Once you get the hang of the sequence, it can be very portable—I had one student who did it against the wall of a ladies room at the airport!

■ **Sun Salute at the Wall**   ■ **Sun Salute at the Chair**

SUN SALUTE AT THE WALL

BENEFITS

Sun Salute can be instrumental in building muscle tone and strength, and helps build energy levels so you can do more activities without becoming tired or short of breath. Your circulation will improve and your body will get better at using oxygen. You may even lose a few pounds! Overall, this sequence done regularly will enhance your self-esteem and make you feel more relaxed and cheerful. Even more important, this simple exercise can slow down the progression of COPD. (See available website for downloadable session in Resource section, page 173).

> **TIP** Prepare for this sequence by placing your mat perpendicular to the edge of the wall. Start by doing only one repetition, and gradually increase up to three rounds.

TECHNIQUE

Stand facing the wall a few more inches that an arm's length away from the wall with the feet about a foot apart, parallel to the sides of your mat.

Inhale: Bring the hands together at the front of the chest. Exhale, and feel yourself connecting with the earth.

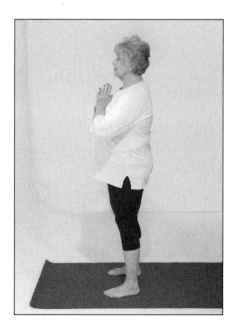

Hands in front of chest

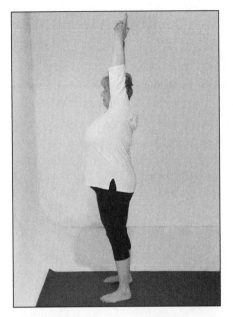

Inhale: On the next inhale, drop the arms to the sides of the body, turn the palms face up, and raise the arms up overhead. The palms will be facing each other, or you can clasp the fingers together.

Arms overhead

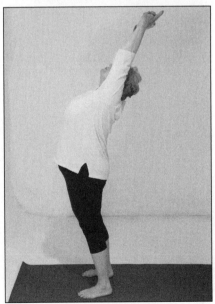

Exhale: Bend back, keeping the arms alongside the ears to protect the neck. Feel the shoulder blades squeezing together rather than the shoulders hiking up toward the ears.

Bend back

Inhale: Come out of your backbend into neutral, arms overhead with fingers locked or separate with palms facing each other.

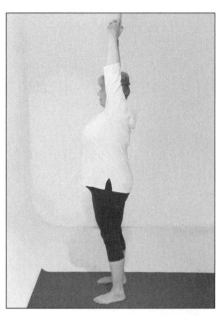

Arms overhead

Exhale: Bend forward from the hips as the arms float out to the sides, in a swan dive motion, then the arms will come to rest hanging alongside the ears. Soften the back of your neck in this standing forward bend.

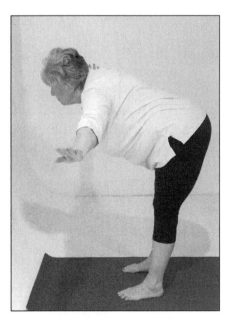

Forward bend

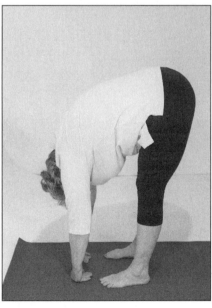

Arms hanging

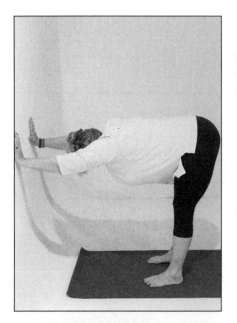

Inhale: Bring the hands up to the wall, about the same level as your hips. We call this the "L" because that is the shape your body will take. Take a few normal breaths here, and notice the side ribs moving in and out with the breath.

Hands up to the wall

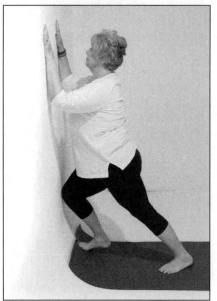

Exhale: Bring the right foot to the edge of the wall, coming into a lunge. Let the knee rest on the wall for support. Bring the forearms and palms to the wall with the upper arms in line with the shoulders. Continue breathing; use pursed lip breathing if you notice you're getting short of breath.

Come into a lunge

Inhale: Step the right foot back to meet the left, as you bring your palms back down to the hip level, returning to the "L" position. Continue in pursed lip breathing.

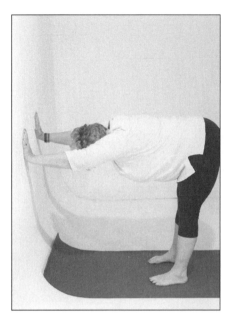

"L" Posiiton

Now we'll do this on the other side—

Exhale: Bring the left foot to the wall, coming into a lunge. Rest the left knee on the wall and allow the right heel to lift off the floor. Forearms and palms come to the wall with the upper arms in line with the shoulders if possible. Square your hips to the wall if you can. Continue to breathe using pursed lips.

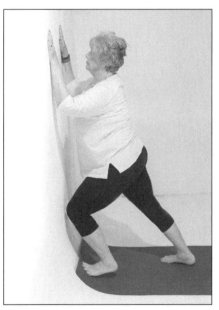

Come into a lunge

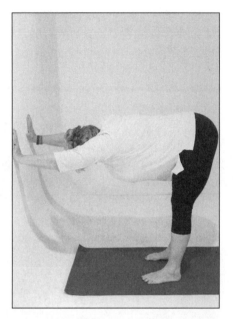

Inhale: Step the left foot back to meet the right, as you bring your palms back down to the hip level, and once again bring the hands up to the wall, about the same level as your hips, returning to the "L." Continue in pursed lip breathing.

"L" Position

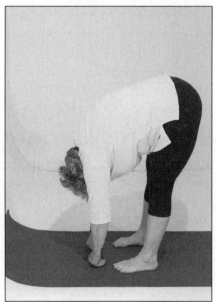

Exhale: Bending at the hips, push away from the wall, and hang down. Let the weight of the head and the arms draw the body down. Soften the knees so there is no strain. Breathe and relax.

Hanging down

Inhale: Bending the knees and coming into a squat bring the arms alongside the head as the face looks toward the floor. Continue moving upward until you're standing tall with the arms overhead, palms facing each other. Feel free to take a few breaths to complete this movement, pausing on the exhale and moving on the inhale.

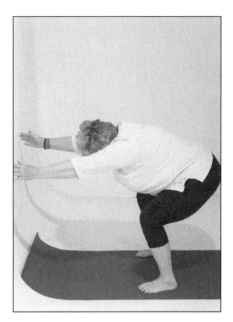

Squat Position

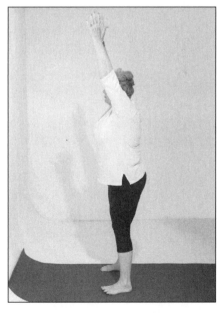

Standing tall

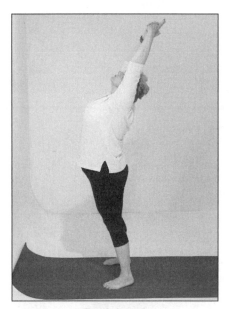

Back bend

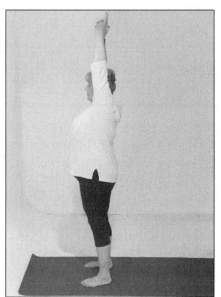

Arms overhead

Exhale: Bring back into a gentle back bend, feeling the squeeze between the shoulder blades.

Inhale: Come out of your back bend with arms straight overhead.

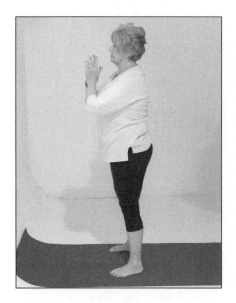

Exhale: To complete the Sun Salute, release the arms out to the sides and down then bring the palms together at the heart center. Close your eyes, if that's comfortable for you. Let the arms come to the sides and adjust your feet. Pause as you continue to breathe through pursed lips and notice the effect of this fantastic sequence.

Arms at heart center

SUN SALUTE AT THE CHAIR

BENEFITS

So many benefits, physiologically! The lunges help strengthen the muscles of the legs.

In addition, the lunges open the torso, providing more space for the internal organs to be refreshed with new blood. The forward bends help lower blood pressure, bring a fresh supply of blood to the brain, and give a gentle massage to the internal organs. The back bends open the chest area, providing more space for the lungs to bring in more oxygen. And the gentle twists massage the organs of digestion, helping to eliminate stagnation. So imagine that the internal organs of the core are like a sponge. We're squeezing out old fluids as we scrunch up (forward bend) and then as we bend back, there's room for fresh blood and other healthy fluids to rush back in, revitalizing us.

Note that we initiate each movement with an inhale or an exhale, but then we continue to breathe in pursed lip breathing as you hold the stretch, as you explore and deepen each pose. A video version of this sequence can be found in the Resource section, page 173, if you prefer to be guided through the sequence.

> **TIP** Place your mat underneath your chair, positioning it so the chair won't slide around. The seat of the chair will be facing away from you. Just do one round when you are starting out, but increase over time to up to three repetitions.

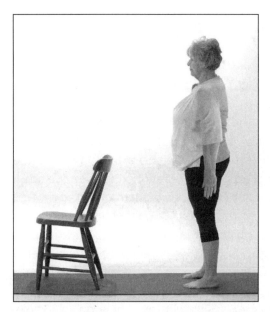

TECHNIQUE

Stand facing the back of your chair, a few more inches than an arm's length away from the top of the chair with the feet about a foot apart, parallel to the sides of your mat.

Facing back of chair

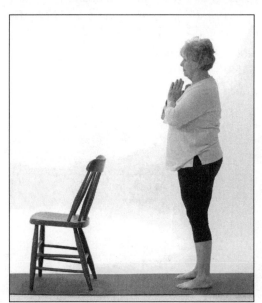

Inhale: Bring the hands together at the front of the chest. Exhale, and feel yourself connecting with the earth.

Hands together

Inhale: On the next inhale, drop the arms to the sides of the body, turn the palms face up, and raise the arms up overhead. The palms will be facing each other, or you can clasp the fingers together.

Arms overhead

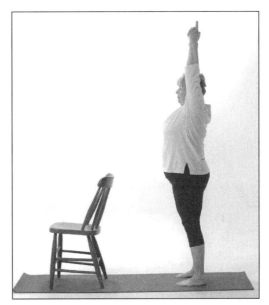

Exhale: Bend back, keeping the arms alongside the ears to protect the neck. Feel the shoulder blades squeezing together.

Inhale: Come out of your backbend into neutral, arms overhead with fingers locked or separate with palms facing each other.

Bend back

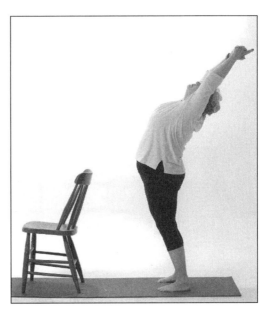

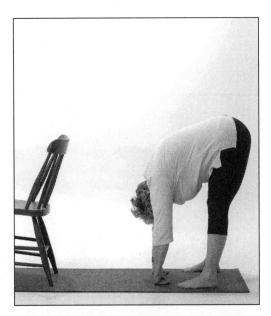

Exhale: Bend forward from the hips as the arms float out to the sides, in a swan dive motion, then the arms will come to rest dangling beside the ears. Soften the back of your neck in this standing forward bend.

Bend forward

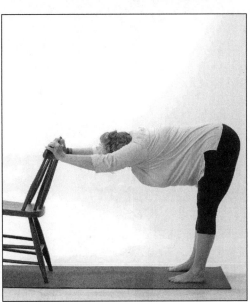

Inhale: Bring the hands to the top of the back of the chair, come into the "L" position, with a flat back. The head is between the arms. Knees can be straight or not—a slight bend is fine. Try to be aware of a softening in the back of the neck. Also, observe your breath expanding the side ribs, and take a few breaths here, ending on an exhalation.

"L" Position

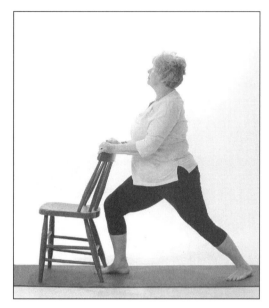

Inhale: Next is a lunge— bring the right foot close to the chair, bending the knee. The hands are holding the top of the chair's back, but keep the shoulders from rising, and tuck the elbows gently towards the torso. The heel of the back leg will lift. Sink into the lunge and breathe normally.

Lunge Position

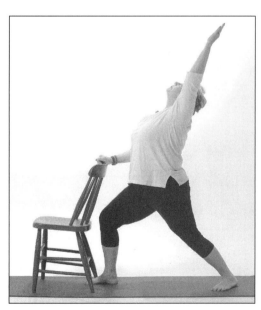

Inhale: Raise the left arm overhead.

Exhale: Bend back, keeping the left arm alongside the head. Breathe normally as you deepen your stretch.

Left arm overhead

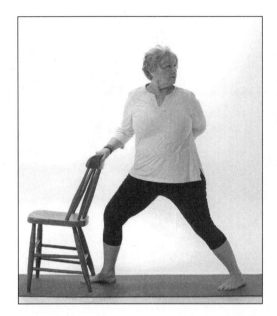

Exhale: Bring the left arm down, as you begin to twist to the left, bringing the left arm around behind the back. Breathe deeply as you focus on your spine.

Left arm behind back

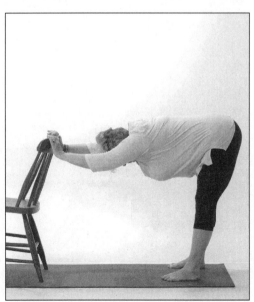

Inhale: Release the twist. Step the right foot back to meet the left, bring the left arm to the chair and come back into the "L," breathing normally.

"L" Position

Now we're going to do the other side!

Inhale: Now lunge on the other side—bring the left foot close to the chair, have the knee bent. Sink deeply into your lunge as you take a breath or two.

Lunge Position

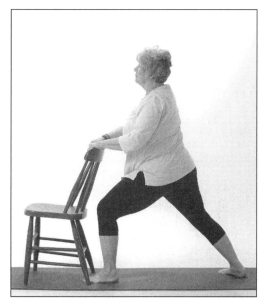

Inhale: Raise the right arm overhead, perpendicular to the floor.

Right arm overhead

Exhale: Gently bend back, keeping the right arm beside the head. Breathe normally expanding the chest.

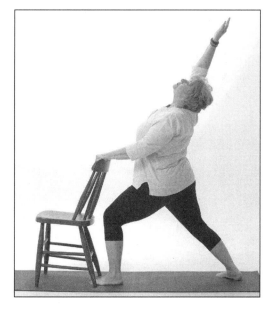

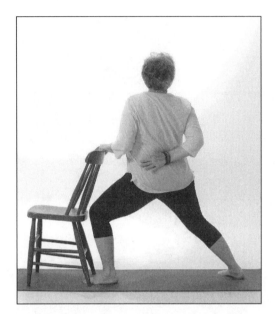

Exhale: Release the back bend, and begin to come into your twist. Bring the right arm behind the back and turn the head looking right. Keep the bottom of the chin parallel to the floor.

Right arm behind back

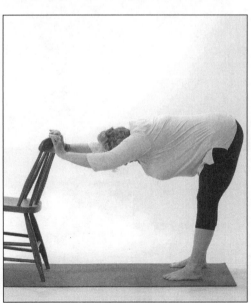

Inhale: Release the twist, slowly and deliberately. Step the front foot back to meet the right foot, coming into the "L" position. Notice the sensations in the body as you breathe deeply into the side ribs, which are well expanded in this pose.

"L" Position

Exhale: Soften the knees and bend forward, allowing the body to hang. You may clasp your elbows and bring the head between the arms or you can allow the arms to hang loosely.

Bend forward

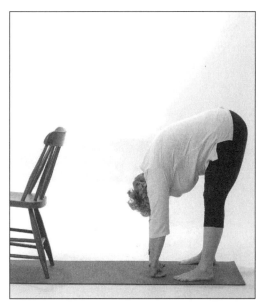

Inhale: Drop the buttocks and come into a squat, extending the arms parallel to the floor, keeping them close to the ears. The head is facing the floor. Take care not to let the knees cave in toward each other. Take a breath or two here before coming up a little higher.

Squat Position

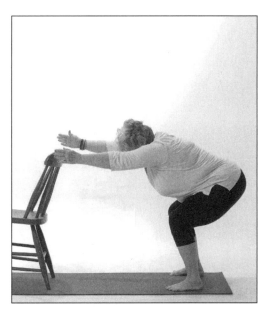

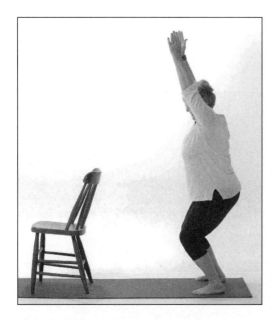

Begin to unbend knees

Inhale: Begin to partially unbend the knees, sweep the arms out and up until you come about three quarters of the way to full standing position. (Sweeping the arms out to bring yourself to standing can be very hard on the spine unless you do the previous step where the body is in the squat.) Keep the arms alongside the ears, and imagine there is a chair behind you that you're about to sit down on. Take care not to let the knees cave in toward each other.

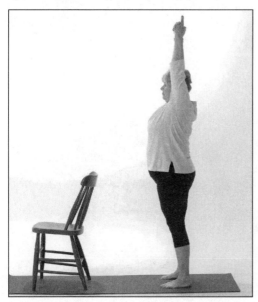

Exhale: Hold chair position for a few breaths, feeling the strength in your legs and the expansiveness in the torso.

Inhale: Straighten the legs, bringing the arms overhead, palms facing each other. Drop your shoulders, please!

Arms overhead

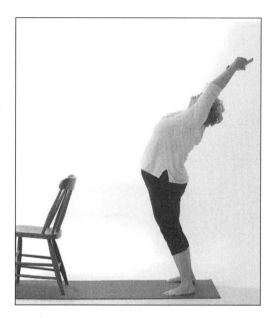

Exhale: Bend back, feeling a squeeze across the shoulder blades.

Bend back

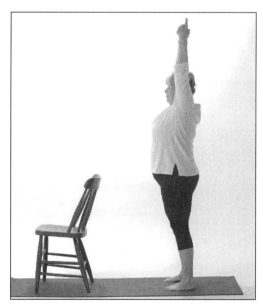

Inhale: Come back to neutral, arms overhead.

Arms overhead

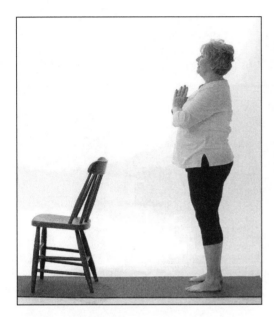

Exhale: Float the arms down, palms facing the earth, until they come to the sides of the body. Bring the palms back together at the heart center, close the eyes. Pause for a moment, then drop the arms, adjust the feet until comfortable, and relax as you observe the effects of your practice.

Palms at heart center

Duration: Take all the time you need with this powerful sequence. Done quickly, it can perk you up when you start to space out in the late afternoon. Or, if you're feeling jumpy and unsettled, this sequence can be done slowly to calm you down.

RESTORATIVE POSES

In the next section, we will explore the delicious sensation of deep rest. Using a variety of props, blankets, sandbag, eye pillows, and soothing music, we give the body and mind a chance to settle into the tranquility of our natural, undisturbed self. Restorative postures help to counteract the effects of the hustle and bustle of everyday life in our busy culture. Each pose works in a passive, not active, way to balance the subtle energies flowing through our bodies. Because these poses are held without moving they allow cortisol levels to drop. When these stress hormones calm down, it brings on the relaxation response.

TIP These exercises can be done lying on the floor on your mat. If you're not comfortable getting down to the floor, try lying on your bed instead. Gather your props: eye pillow, bolsters or pillows, blankets, and sandbag. Turn on some quiet music to listen to, helping you to relax. I created a CD that mimics the timing of the routines so I know when to come out of one pose exercise and move into the next. See Resource section, page 173.

- Torso Opener
- Heart Opener
- Hip Elevation
- Leg Elevation
- Dead to the World

TORSO OPENER

BENEFITS

This exercise opens the chest up to allow for deeper breathing. It helps to counteract the tendency we have for hunching the shoulders forward, as we sit at our computers or phones. It helps improve digestion and is beneficial for the female organs, making it a tonic for women whether you are menstruating, pregnant, or going through menopause.

TECHNIQUE

Begin to set up your props, starting with 2 blocks at the top of your mat. One block will be horizontal and one vertical. Move your bolster so it lies on the blocks with the highest part at the head of your

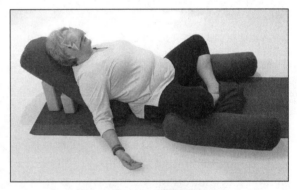

Torso Opener Position

mat. Place your buttocks at the bottom end of the bolster and lie back onto the bolster. (This may require some skill—sometimes the blocks fall over!) If you're able, bend the knees and place the soles of the feet together, allowing the knees to fall to the side. Drape a sandbag across the feet and an eye pillow on the eyes. You may want to place additional bolsters or pillows under the knees for comfort. If this isn't available to you, simply extend the legs out in front of you, placing a bolster under the knees if you like. Notice the feeling of openness in the low belly and imagine that with each inhalation, you are bringing fresh energy to that area. Allow stagnant energy to flow out of the body with the exhalations.

Duration: Enjoy a 10 to 15 minute relaxation in this position. When you're ready to come out, remove the sandbag, take the bolsters under the knees to the side, and remove the blocks. Take care to come out of the position gently as you begin to bring your awareness back to reality!

HEART OPENER

BENEFITS

Another chest opener, this position helps bring fresh energy throughout the body and creates a feeling of freedom in the sternum, lungs, and heart.

TECHNIQUE

You'll need 2 bolsters for the torso and a pillow for under the head. Place one bolster under the knees and another under the mid-back area. Place a pillow under the head for a head rest. Extend the arms out in a T-shape, between the head rest and the upper body bolster. If that's not comfortable, use a small bolster or a rolled up blanket. Once you have a comfortable posture, add your eye pillow.

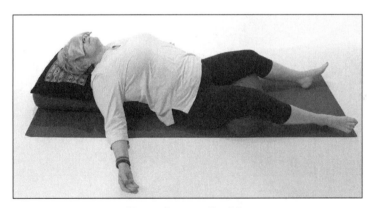

Chest Opener Position

Duration: Relax in this position for 5 to 15 minutes. Notice the gentle rising and falling of the belly as you focus on your breathing. When ready to come out of the position, remove the mid-back bolster, and move the other one a little further down your mat. Remove the head-rest and eye pillow.

HIP ELEVATION

BENEFITS

This routine helps to reverse the flow of blood and lymph from their normal direction, refreshing the lymph and bringing a fresh supply of blood to the brain.

TECHNIQUE

Only one prop is needed—a bolster. Slide the bolster you have at your feet from the last position up and under your buttocks. Bend the knees and place the feet under the knees, about a foot apart. Lift the hips to rest them back onto the bolster. Extend the arms out to the sides and relax into the position. Add the eye pillow if you like, and you can also add the sandbag on the belly.

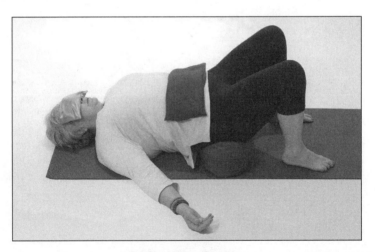

Hip Elevation Position

Duration: Rest easy in this position for 5 to 15 minutes. When you're ready to move again, remove the eye pillow and sandbag and gently roll off the bolster.

LEG ELEVATION

BENEFITS

Here's another routine that helps to move stagnant energy. With the legs up over the head, it allows spent blood to drain, with the help of gravity, back to the lungs for re-oxygenation. The lymph gets moved as well, helping to improve your immune system.

TECHNIQUE

At the wall: Find a wall that is free of pictures and furniture. Sit alongside the wall with the legs outstretched, parallel to the wall. Begin to fall back (carefully) until the legs come up to the wall, allowing the extended legs to rest against the wall. Try to scooch your cheeks right up to the wall so you're not crooked. Get comfortable, placing an eye pillow on your eyes and even a sandbag on the feet.

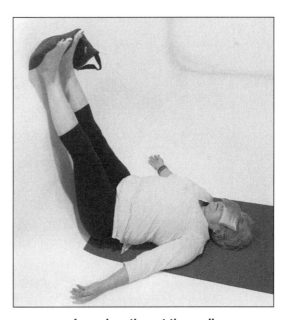

Leg elevation at the wall

Duration: Stay here for up to 10 minutes. If the legs get restless, bend the knees and slide the feet down the wall, about half way to your bottom. Then, after a minute or so, extend the legs up the wall again. When you're ready to come out of the position, remove the sandbag and lower both legs together, sliding them down the wall. Bend the knees and come into a fetal position while you begin to get your wits about you before coming up to a seated posture.

At the chair: Lying on your mat with the chair facing you, place your hands on the floor behind you so you can bend the knees, bringing the legs up so the calves rest on the chair. Rest the eye pillow on the eyes and the sandbag on the belly. Notice if there's any part of the body that's holding on to tension and gently release.

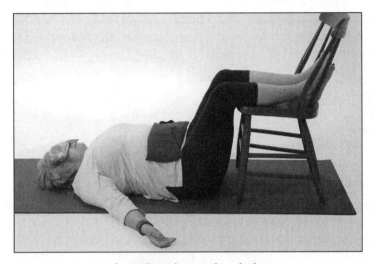

Leg elevation at the chair

Duration: Stay here for about 10 minutes. If the legs get restless, extend the legs up toward the ceiling, one at a time if necessary. Make circles with the ankles or point and flex the feet. Then bring each leg back so the calf rests on the seat of the chair. When you're ready to come out of the position, remove the eye pillow and sandbag then gently roll to the side before coming to a seated posture.

At the bed: Place your mat perpendicular to your bed. Sit down sideways on the mat and swing the legs up to the top of the mattress, lowering the upper body to lie down on the mat. Use whatever props make you feel comfortable.

Duration: Stay in this restful position for about 10 minutes. When you're ready to come out of the position, gently fall to the side and rest in fetal position until you're ready to sit up.

DEAD TO THE WORLD

BENEFITS

In this routine you don't have to do anything but relax. It gives the body a chance to assimilate the benefits of the work we've done, whether it's the flexibility routine, the standing exercises, or the restorative routines. Corpse or Dead To The World position helps the body to remember what it feels like to be deeply relaxed, allowing the body to "right" itself. When done on a regular basis, adding the body scan that we'll talk about shortly, corpse pose promotes healing throughout the body and mind.

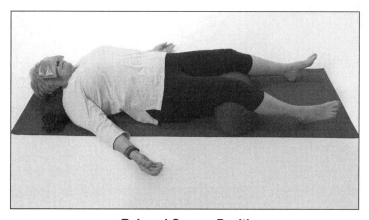

Relaxed Corpse Position

TECHNIQUE

This routine can be done seated in a chair, lying on the floor on your mat, or lying on your bed. Wear loose clothing with a stretchy waist and have a blanket or sweater handy, as we will be resting for quite a long time and you may find yourself getting chilly. Once you lie down, have the feet spread about a foot (or more, based on what feels the most comfortable), let the arms be about a foot away from the sides of the body, palms up. Place a bolster under the knees if you need it and a small tootsie roll pillow under the neck as well. Bring the eye pillow to the eyes. Feel that the floor is doing all the work of supporting your body, there is no effort needed.

Bring the awareness to the breath, and enjoy a few gentle breaths. If you only have a short amount of time, continue to focus on the breath for 3 to 7 minutes. Enjoy the bliss of letting go and etch that feeling into your mind so you can remember to come back to this feeling anytime you begin to stress out.

You now have several options for getting more comfortable in your own body, through the exercises of stretching, bending, twisting, bowing, and resting. In the next chapter we offer even more ways of improving your body awareness, through the practice of breathing techniques. When we take control of the breath, automatically the mind will follow and become more calm, an essential tool to have when feeling short of breath.

Chapter 8

Breathing Techniques

Now that you've warmed up the body with some stretching exercises, you're ready for the practice of controlling and expanding the breath. In this chapter, we will offer a handful of breathing techniques that will help build your strength, your energy level, and your peace of mind. You may have already been aware that when you are concentrating deeply on something, your breath almost stops. Conversely, when you are excited or frightened your breath speeds up which can exacerbate the challenge of having COPD. The various breathing practices I'm about to show you will give you more control over the body's natural reaction to events. They come from an ancient tradition and have worn the test of time. The following breathing practices will change your life, however check with your physician regarding any breathing exercises to make sure they are safe for you. So let's begin!

- Diaphragmatic Breath
- Alternate Nostril Breath
- Bellows Breath
- Humming Bee Breath

Advanced Breathing Techniques

- Cooling Breath
- Wheezing Breath
- Hissing Breath

DIAPHRAGMATIC BREATH

BENEFITS

This simple three-part breath is the cornerstone of all the breathing exercises. It helps open the chest and bring awareness to the breathing mechanism.

TECHNIQUE

Sit comfortably with feet on the floor or a pillow. Sit forward on your chair and keep your spine long and your shoulders wide. Close the eyes, and begin to watch the breath. The action of the belly should be:

On the inhale, the belly expands, the way a balloon expands when you fill it up with air.

On the exhale, the belly collapses, as if you had let all the air out of a balloon.

The three-parts of the breathing capacity are:

1. The abdomen

2. The rib cage or middle chest

3. The upper chest

Begin to fill up the belly with air, feel it expand, and then exhale slowly, quietly, and with control. Repeat this a few more times, keeping the focus just on the belly.

Next begin to fill the belly and then the rib cage, expanding the breath from the bottom of the lungs and moving upwards. Exhale from the rib cage, then from the belly and repeat a few times.

Finally, fill the belly, rib cage, and the upper chest with air. Now the lungs are fully expanded. You may feel the collarbones rise slightly, but don't let the shoulders creep up too. The exhalation starts at the top of the lungs, goes through the mid-section, and finally the belly empties and is drawn in toward the spine. Try using pursed lip breathing on the exhale. This constitutes one round.

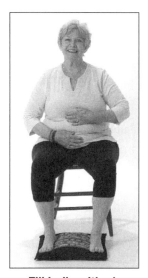
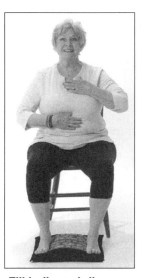
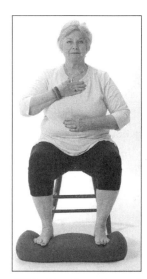

| **Fill belly with air and release** | **Fill belly and rib cage and release** | **Fill belly, rib cage, and upper chest and release** |

Duration: Begin with just a few rounds. Over time, increase the number of rounds to 7 to 10 rounds.

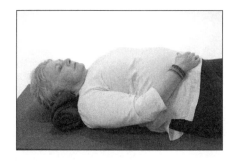

Gentle rising and falling of abdomen with each breath

Consideration: If you find that your belly is going in on the inhalation and out on the exhalation, you might be doing reverse breathing. To retrain your body and change your breathing habits, try doing this practice while lying comfortably on your bed. Place one hand on the abdomen and watch the gentle rising and falling with each breath. With practice, this will be so natural to you that you can do it sitting up too.

BELLOWS BREATH

BENEFITS

Next is the bellows breath, is also known as "mental floss," because it is especially beneficial for the brain. It really helps to perk you up in mid-afternoon when you might reach for another cup of coffee or a cocktail. And no negative side effects! It helps to re-oxygenate the blood and remove toxins that may have been dumped into the bloodstream from your exercises.

TECHNIQUE

Sit comfortably with your spine long and your shoulders wide but relaxed. Begin with a few rounds of the basic three-part breath (see page 93). After the final exhale, inhale only into the low belly with a short inhalation. Then, with a snap of the abdomen, pull your belly into the spine and force your breath out through your nostrils. Imagine you are trying to blow a feather off your nose. Continue with short inhalations into your belly and quick, forceful exhalations. After the last round, finish with a full three-part inhale and a long exhale through pursed lips (see page 94).

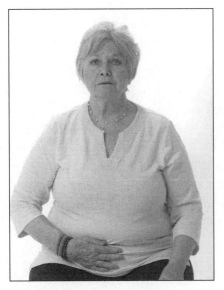
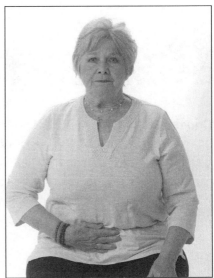

Inhale into low belly   **Breathe out through nostrils**

Duration: Begin with 3 to 5 repetitions, increasing over time to up to twenty to constitute one round. Do one to three rounds, as you increase your capacity.

Consideration: The short snap of the exhale requires the same force used to blow your nose, so have a tissue handy! If you begin to feel dizzy, stop and take a break. As mentioned, check with your physician regarding this and any other breathing exercises to make sure they are safe for you.

ALTERNATE NOSTRIL BREATH

BENEFITS

The alternate nostril breath is very calming to the nervous system and is often practiced before a meditation session. It helps to balance the right and left brain and has a relaxing effect on the mind; it helps to alleviate stress. It may also alleviate hypertension as the practice stimulates various nerves that reach different areas of the hypothalamus, a part of the brain that helps to regulate blood pressure.

TECHNIQUE

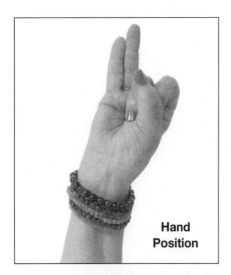

Hand Position

After getting settled in your comfortable posture, using your right hand make a gentle fist and then extend your thumb, pinky, and ring finger. Tuck your right elbow close to your chest and bring your thumb close to your right nostril. Inhale through both nostrils, then block off your right nostril with your thumb as you exhale out of the left nostril, using the simple three-part breath (see page 93). Inhale through your left nostril and then block it off with your extended pinky and ring finger, removing your thumb from your right nostril so that you can exhale from it. Inhale right, exhale left. Continue in this pattern, switching nostrils after each inhalation. Gradually, you will notice the exhalations getting longer than the inhalations. This is a good thing, as it allows the oxygen to stay in your body longer, increasing your vitality. The exhalations can be up to twice as long as the inhalations. Finish with an exhalation out of your right nostril. Bring your hands to your lap and take a moment to feel the peaceful effect of this practice.

Begin by taking a breath through both nostrils. Then proceed to follow the photographs below.

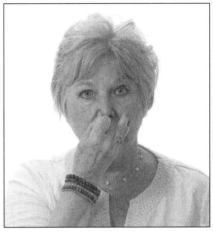

1. Thumb closes right nostril, exhale left

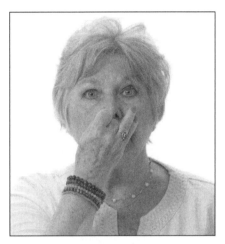

2. Block right nostril, inhale

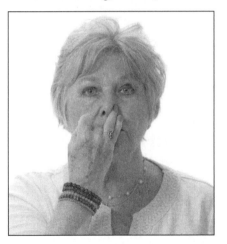

3. Fingers close left nostril, exhale right

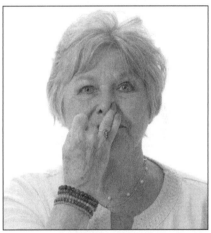

4. Block left nostril, inhale right and then repeat from number 1 above

Duration: Practice the nerve purifying breath for one to three minutes.

Consideration: Don't strain as you lengthen the exhalations. Keep the breath soft and fluid each time you switch nostrils. Although these breathing techniques have been shown to lower blood pressure, you should not forego medication or conventional treatment for hypertension without first consulting your doctor.

HUMMING BEE BREATH

BENEFITS

The humming bee breath provides a real experience of bliss. It is a soothing practice, ideal for promoting sleep and alleviating depression. It strengthens the voice and eliminates throat ailments, and has been proven to speed up healing. The humming bee breath can be used instead of the nerve purifying breath as a preparation for meditation. It's also just fun to do!

TECHNIQUE

Sit comfortably, with your spine long and your shoulders wide. Close your eyes and do two or three rounds of the simple three-part breath (see page 93). When you are ready, inhale deeply through the nostrils and, with your teeth slightly separated and lips gently closed, begin humming as you exhale. Continue to hum, smoothly and evenly, at any pitch, until all the air is expelled. Observe the pleasant buzzing in your head and imagine the vibrations going straight up through the crown of your head and out into the universe. When you run out of breath, you have completed one round and can inhale again. Allow your mind to become absorbed by the humming sound.

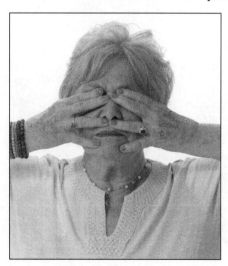

Humming Bee Position

Duration: Do five rounds of the humming bee breath, at various pitches, without opening your eyes. Once you've finished, sit quietly and listen. You should hear the humming continuing inside you. As you become better attuned to this subtle humming, it can help you access the deep peace of your true nature.

ADVANCED BREATHING PRACTICES

The following practices are for more experienced practitioners and may need the approval of your health care professionals before you begin practicing.

COOLING BREATH

BENEFITS

Cooling breath is a breathing technique that helps to keep you cool, and is best used in warmer weather.

TECHNIQUE

Using the same gentle three-part breathing technique mentioned earlier, curl your tongue into a cylindrical shape, making it like a straw. Inhale into the "straw," which cools the breath, close the mouth and hold the breath briefly if you're able. Exhale slowly out of the nostrils or through pursed lips. This is one round.

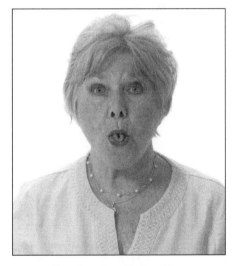

Duration: Try one to five repetitions of this cooling breath.

Consideration: This is not recommended for people with asthma, untreated low blood pressure, or bronchitis.

Cooling Breath Position

WHEEZING BREATH

BENEFITS

This breath cools the body, purifies and stimulates the gums, and also helps wake you up if you're sleepy. In addition, it may quench your thirst and even assuage hunger! I use it during the fall allergy season, when my nose gets stuffed up and my regular breathing practices are difficult to do. It's helpful as a stress management tool because it brings your awareness back to your breathing, increases energy in the system, and cleans the subtle nerve currents similar to the meridians used in acupuncture. It also helps to cool excited emotions and relieve mental tensions.

TECHNIQUE

Sit comfortably, with your spine long and your shoulders wide. Close your eyes and become aware of your breath, allowing it to slow down and become more rhythmic. After a minute or two, bare your teeth and curl your tongue back so that it touches the soft palate on the roof of your mouth. You should look like you're wearing a wide, maniacal grin. Inhale through your teeth, making a wet, slurpy sound. You will feel a coolness

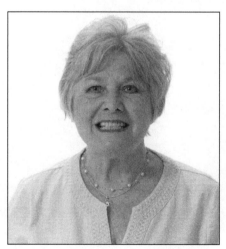

Wheezing Breath Position

as the air enters the sides of your mouth. Hold the breath for a few seconds, close your mouth, and then exhale slowly out of your nostrils.

Duration: Do as many repetitions as comfortable for you, up to 8.

Consideration: This is not recommended for people with asthma, untreated low blood pressure, or bronchitis.

Don't worry about trying to master all these techniques. We're just including them to offer some variety. If you are comfortable doing the three-part breath and want to stick with that, that's fine—the important thing is to practice every day, ideally for 20 minutes.

HISSING BREATH

BENEFITS

In the breathing exercises, the longer you are able to exhale, the greater the benefits to your system. A slow exhalation helps your body distribute energy into the most subtle areas of the body—the cells, and even the spaces between the cells! One way to prolong your exhalations is through the hissing breath. This practice helps calm your mind and focus restless thoughts. It also increases circulation to your throat and improves digestion and respiratory problems.

TECHNIQUE

Sit comfortably, with your spine long and your shoulders wide. Begin by closing your eyes and mouth and relaxing your entire body. Take some time to watch your breath, allowing it to gradually slow down and become more rhythmic. Inhale, bringing your awareness to your throat and as you exhale slowly partially contract the glottis muscles at the back of your throat. This will create a gentle hissing sound, so subtle that only you will be able to hear it. It's the same sound that a sleeping baby makes, almost like a soft snore. Another way to ensure that you are doing a hissing breath correctly is to first open your mouth and hiss like an angry cat. Now try the same hiss, closing your mouth and your glottis. After you have inhaled and exhaled once in this manner, you have completed a round.

Duration: Do only as many as comfortable, up to 5 rounds.

Consideration: This exercise is not recommended for beginners. Avoid straining your throat by slowly building up to a longer practice over time.

MEDITATION AND VISUALIZATION

For someone with breathing challenges, meditation can be key to calming the mind when experiencing breathlessness. Imagine that the peacefulness of your true inner self is like a beautiful blue sky on a summer day. The thoughts that come from the mind are like the clouds that may float across the clear blue sky, sometimes decorating the sky and other times obscuring the blue sky completely.

In meditation we focus on the sky, and disregard the clouds, which in our analogy, have no power to change the beauty of the clear blue sky. Yes, clouds may appear, but we don't have to get involved with them. We don't have to analyze the thoughts that pop into the mind, or figure anything out during our meditation time. We simply observe whatever thoughts arise and go back to focusing on whatever you have chosen as the focal point of your meditation.

With regular practice, meditation helps you to reconnect with your inner peace, making it easier to return to that state when we get upset or feel nervous that we might run out of breath. There are many techniques that can bring you into that state of tranquility—I'll offer a few different approaches. If none of these approaches appeals to you, check out the visualizations that are offered later in this chapter.

- **So Hum Meditation**

- **Mantra Meditation**

- **Visualizations**

- **Progressive Deep Relaxation**

SO HUM MEDITATION

BENEFITS

This meditation calms the mind, is helpful for insomnia and heart disease, and creates inner stability. And it's portable. Whether you're in your car or on the subway,

TECHNIQUE

It's best to meditate on an empty stomach so that you're more alert. Sit on a comfortable chair with your feet on the floor. Loosen your tie and your belt. Take off your shoes if possible. If you're comfortable sitting forward on the chair, that's ideal—you want your back to be long and straight rather than slumping back into the chair. Let the shoulders be relaxed but open. Let the hands rest softly on the thighs. Make a vow that you won't move a single muscle during your session. It is helpful to select a regular time each day to have your meditation session and do your best to stick to your schedule.

Close and soften the eyes. Begin simple three-part breathing using pursed lips if that's comfortable for you. (See page 94.) Notice the breath as it enters the body— it's a little cool. As the breath leaves the body, notice that it feels warmer. Now listen to the sound of the breath. When it comes into the nostrils, it makes a sound, *so.* As you exhale, the sound changes a little to sound like *hum,* or if you're using pursed lips, it may sound like *fooo.*

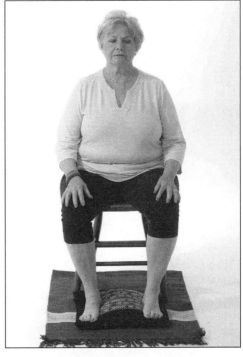

Sitting Meditation Position

159

TIP Don't be discouraged when the mind wanders off to think about the latest episode of your favorite TV show. Or you may start to worry that you left the lights on in the kitchen. The mind is always looking for a chore! Noticing that the mind has wandered away from the breath is the first step in meditating.

Duration: Try to stay focused on these sounds as you continue to breathe gently, up to 10 minutes. Over time you can increase your meditation up to 30 minutes. When you're ready to come back to regular consciousness, open the eyes slowly and take time to observe your surroundings. Notice how calm you feel, and bring that calmness into your life, into your work, into your family. The world needs all the tranquility you can bring to it.

Walking to the office or doing the dishes, you can always observe your breath.

MANTRA MEDITATION

BENEFITS

Another classic meditation technique is sacred word, or mantra meditation. The word mantra comes from the word for mind, indicating that it's a tool for training the mind. The ancient Sanskrit mantras are sound formulas that are used to elevate the mind at a subtle vibratory level. For our purposes, we will use a short affirmation, such as "I am Love," or "All is well." But once you select a mantra, use the same one every time you meditate, rather than changing it every session. Your chosen mantra will become more powerful the more you use it, bringing you into a deeper state of peace.

TECHNIQUE

Wait a couple hours after a big meal so that you don't fall asleep as you're digesting! Come into your comfortable sitting position on your chair with feet on the floor or a bolster. Unbuckle your belt or pants so you're completely at ease. Have the eyes closed and soft inside the eye sockets. Begin to silently repeat your chosen mantra. It won't be long before the mind wanders away and starts thinking about other pressing thoughts. Don't worry, simply return to the mantra when you become aware of the mind's wandering. With regular practice, the mind will begin to settle more easily and you'll enjoy the peaceful stillness within.

Duration: As a beginner, try to sit steadily for 10 minutes twice a day. Gradually increase the time of your meditation to 30 minutes, twice a day. Come out of your meditation by gently opening the eyes, having a stretch, and observing the shift in your consciousness.

VISUALIZATIONS

If you have a creative nature or a restless mind, instead of trying to meditate, it can be helpful to engage the mind with a task. Instead of perseverating on your to-do list, which can increase anxiety, we give the mind a task of following a script that will keep the mind focused on more positive images. The following script focuses on the five senses, giving the mind a pleasurable alternative to its habit of worrying. Check out the resource section for a downloadable audio file of the script. This first visualization is designed for anyone challenged with COPD.

BENEFITS

As you begin to experience the "air hunger" common to COPD patients, it's helpful to practice this visualization to calm the body and mind. It will reduce muscle tension in the neck, chest, and throat, allowing the breath to become relaxed as well. This visualization will also reduce inflammation in the airways. The more regularly you practice, the faster you'll feel relief.

The Meaning of Mantra

The word *mantra* has become part of our current vernacular, and as is often the case, has lost its original meaning. The mantras that I offer in this section derive from a more classical meaning of mantra, namely "sound formula." When we say or chant "Om shanthi," we are aware of its meaning—peace—but on a more subtle level we can perceive a feeling of peace. The mantra embodies peace itself. When we use a mantra for meditation, we embody the quality of the mantra—we bring peace into existence in our very selves. There are thousands of mantras from an ancient time when words had more power. Ancient words from other traditions, such as Amen, Alleluia, Allah hu Akbar, Shalom have a similar effect. Although English affirmations, such as "All is love," are helpful to calm the mind when repeated as the object of meditation, they lack the mystical vibratory element of a classic mantra.

TECHNIQUE

Choose a safe space in which to practice, either sitting on a chair or lying down on the floor or bed. Make sure your clothes aren't restricting you in any way. Begin to make yourself comfortable, while still keeping the spine long and the shoulders relaxed and open. Close and soften the eyes in the sockets. Relax the skin on the face. Relax the neck, the arms, the torso. Feel your buttocks and legs getting heavy. Relax your feet. Now your body is soft and relaxed. Your breathing is becoming slower and quieter and you have plenty of air in your lungs to be perfectly comfortable.

Begin to imagine your lungs in your mind's eye. Visualize them expanding and contracting with each breath. Imagine the alveoli (air sacs) releasing spent air with every exhalation. Take a moment to hold that image. Then, can you also imagine the sweet fragrance of your favorite flower? Pause as you concentrate on that sensation. Then engage your sense of touch by imagining a soft breeze wafting across your body. Pause as you focus on that sensation. Now engage your sense of taste by imagining your favorite treat. Imagine a bite of chocolate, or a delicious ripe mango—whatever you enjoy. Can you taste it, on your mind's tongue? Pause as you enjoy the sensation of deliciousness. Next, move your awareness to your inner hearing—can you hear a beautiful melody, audiating a tune you know, or perhaps making one up on the spot? Listen deeply. Now bring your awareness to an image of serenity. Perhaps it's a beach at sunset. Or picture a scene where the sun is coming up over a beautiful ripe field of wheat.

Begin to observe the overall sensation of relaxation that is a result of this visualization. Your body and breath and mind are completely relaxed. Enjoy this state of tranquility for a little longer. Then gently begin to breathe a little more deeply, have a stretch, maybe a little yawn as you begin to come back to regular consciousness. When you're ready, open the eyes and take this precious gift of peace into your day, into your life.

PROGRESSIVE DEEP RELAXATION

If you have more time, let me recommend a progressive deep relaxation. In this practice, we tense and relax all the parts of the body, squeezing out any residual tensions. Then we go over the body again mentally, without moving a single muscle. We mentally assess all the parts of the body to see if there are hidden tensions that we can let go of, mentally. The mind and body are at rest, but not asleep in the normal sense. The process of going deeper into stillness allows the body to heal.

BENEFITS

The deep relaxation reduces stress in the muscles and the organs, and helps stabilize the parasympathetic nervous system—the part of the nervous system that controls certain bodily functions, including arousal, digestion, heart rate, and defecation. A regular practice can alleviate symptoms of anxiety that can cause difficulty breathing. As the muscles begin to relax during this technique, automatically the breath will relax as well making it an ideal remedy for shortness of breath experienced in an asthma attack.

TECHNIQUE

Begin by sitting on a chair, lying on the floor, or lying on your bed.

Close the door so that you won't be interrupted.

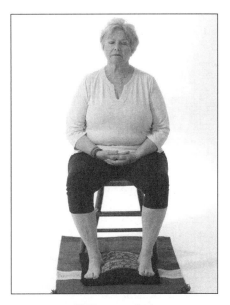

Sitting on chair

Focus your attention on your **right leg**—stretch it out, lift it a couple of inches from the floor and point your toes. Squeeze your right leg tight and then suddenly relax, letting your leg drop as if it were a branch cut from a tree. Roll your leg gently from side to side—and then forget about it. Repeat with your **left leg**.

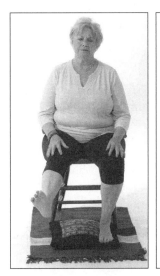
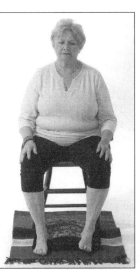
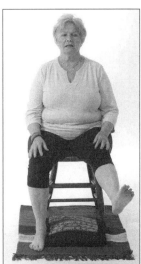

Lift right leg   **Leg dropped to floor**   **Lift left leg**

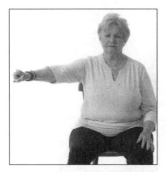 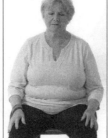 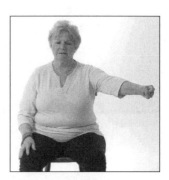

Stretch right arm   **Arms relaxed**   **Stretch left arm**

Continue in the same manner with your **right arm**. Stretch out the fingers on your **right hand** and tighten your whole arm, lifting it a few inches off the ground. Make a fist and squeeze it tight. Make your arm longer and tighter, and then relax, dropping your arm to your lap or the floor.

Roll your right arm gently from side to side, and then forget about it. Shift your attention to your **left arm**, and repeat the process.

Move on to your **buttocks**: squeeze them tight, almost as if you're about to rise right up off the chair. Then release the tension. Shift your focus to your **belly**. Inhale deeply, as if you were filling a big balloon.

Take in as much air as you can hold, letting your belly stick all the way out. Hold your breath in your belly for a moment, then open your mouth and let the air gush out.

Inhale again, this time into your **upper chest**; hold briefly, then open your mouth and exhale.

Now observe your **shoulders**. Shrug them up toward your ears, squeeze them tight, then release. Next, bring your shoulders forward, as if to make them touch under your chin. Squeeze, then let your shoulders drop.

Now move on to your face. Open
your mouth, stick out your tongue,
stretch out all the muscles of your
face, and then release.

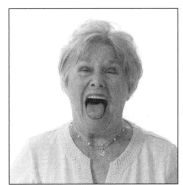

Thrust tongue

Now make a prune face, tightening
all your facial muscles, and then
release.

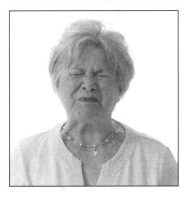

Prune face

Gently roll or turn your **head** from side to side once or twice releasing
any tension in your neck. Then bring your head back to its normal, central
position.

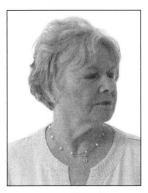 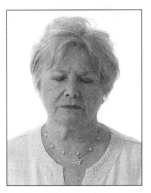 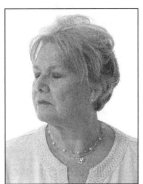

Left side   **Central position**   **Right side**

Take a moment to observe your body, and make any minor adjustments to your position.

You might need to scratch your nose, wiggle the shoulders, or widen the stance of your legs for greater comfort. Mentally check your body and make sure that you aren't holding tension anywhere. You are going to go over your body again, this time without moving a single muscle, so if you feel you need to make an adjustment, do it now. You don't want to keep adjusting throughout the next bit of the process.

You'll be deepening your relaxation mentally, beginning at your feet. Check the bottoms of your feet for any residual tension, and let it melt away. Check your toes. If there is any tension there, gently release it. Continue in this way, relaxing the tops of your feet, your arches, heels, and ankles. Then move into your legs, relaxing your shins, calves, knees, backs of your knees, and thighs. Move your awareness to your hands, forearms, and upper arms. If you find any rebellious muscle that is holding on, let it go. Relax your buttocks, hips, and groin. Relax your belly, rib cage, upper chest, and all your internal organs. Observe the back of your body and relax your spine, shoulder blades, shoulders, and neck. Relax all the parts of your head, from the jaw up to the crown of your head. Relax your lips, tongue, nose, and eyes. Relax your eyebrows and the space between your eyebrows. Relax your ears and temples. Relax.

Take a moment to observe the peaceful feeling in your body. Make note of it so you can refer to this feeling any time you start to notice yourself tensing up. Then observe your breath for a minute or two. Your breath will have become very quiet, almost imperceptible. Don't try to change or control it, just watch. Pause here as you observe your breath. Then move your attention to your mind. Notice how your mind feels very still and quiet, too. Whenever thoughts arise, just let them float away; don't get too interested in them. Become a witness to your mind. Rest easy; stay in this restful state for another 5 or 10 minutes before waking your body. Try not to fall asleep.

To wake your body, begin by bringing your mind back. Gradually deepen your breaths, and your body will naturally want to wake up. Take all the time you need. Gently bring your body back to an active state, wiggling your fingers and toes, and having a nice stretch, as if you've just had a power nap. When you're ready, open the eyes. Take a moment to reorient yourself before your get up from your chair or bed. Take care not to disturb the peaceful feeling that is a result of your practice.

Duration: Try to allow at least 20 to 30 minutes for this rejuvenating practice.

Consideration: Instead of memorizing all the steps, many people find it useful to listen to a recording of instructions, see Resource section page 173.

In this chapter, you have been given a wide variety of practices that you can use to increase vitality and the joy of being alive. The breathing exercises will give you tools for when you begin to feel breathless. An ongoing practice of meditation or visualization will give you more mental clarity and peace of mind, which can be essential in combating the nervousness and panic that is common for someone with breathing challenges. I hope you begin today to use these practices and Take a Deep Breath!

Conclusion

If you're struggling with any kind of breathing challenge, you may have lost faith in your body, in its ability to move comfortably without breathlessness. You may have become afraid to use your body in the way it was designed to move because your illness has restricted you. You may have given up on yourself. It is my hope and prayer that this book will help you better understand your disease and give you tools to begin the process of repairing your relationship to your lungs, to your body overall, and to your emotions.

When researching lung disease previous to writing this book, I discovered something powerful that I think will help you. That is—the lungs have redundancy! That means that, even though you may have damage in parts of your lungs, there are other parts of your lungs that you can begin to "wake up" with the simple and gentle breathing practices we offer. Key to this regeneration is that you begin to practice on a regular basis.

I understand that you are busy with all the chores and errands that are part of life in these busy times, but if you commit to practice pursed lip breathing for 20 minutes every day you will begin to feel better. If you add to that some of the more physical exercises that are offered here, your vitality will increase. And if you allow yourself the delicious experience of restorative routines and deep relaxation and meditation, you will become familiar with a deep peace.

Don't beat yourself up if you have a hard time getting started with a regular practice. It takes tremendous will power to make changes in our life, even when we know it's for the best. I've wanted to have an uninterrupted practice of daily meditation for many years, and I still have periods of intermittent falling off the schedule. But I keep going back to the daily formal practice because that's what I've committed to. Because I know from experience that being regular in my meditation practice can keep me on an even keel, even when life throws some heavy weather at me! Similarly, your daily breathing practice will enable you to increase your body's capacity for oxygen, resulting in a more stress free life, full of vitality and ease.

This book lays it all out for you—now it's in your hands. It's not that complicated. If you think that you have to do all the exercises every day, you might never get started, so be content to do at least 20 to 30 minutes of your favorite practice every day. Mix it up if you get bored with one practice and try something else. Take it easy, not lazy, and you will see the changes!

Resources

This book has a wide range of information on breathing exercises and meditation, but if you would like to learn more about these subjects, or find out more about how these exercises can have a positive effect on your health, this resource section is helpful. In it you will find recommended reading materials, DVDs, CDs, and websites. And this is only a small sample of what is available in bookstores, online, and at your local library.

RECOMMENDED READING

If you would like to further explore any of the subjects covered in *Take a Deep Breath*, I recommend reading the following books. Almost all of the following titles can be found and purchased on Amazon.com.

Agarwal, D., et al, "Assessment for efficacy of additional breathing exercises over improvement in health impairment due to asthma assessed using St. George's respiratory questionnaire," *Int J Yoga*, 2017 Sep–Dec

Behera, D., *Assoc Physicians India*, 1998

Caponigro, Andy, "The Miracle of Breath" , The World Library 2005

Fouladbakhsh, J., et al, "A pilot study of the feasibility and outcomes of yoga for lung cancer survivors," *ONF*, 2014. 41(2), 162–174

Kaminsky, D.A., "Effect of yoga breathing (pranayama) on exercise tolerance in patients with chronic obstructive pulmonary disease: a randomized, controlled trial, *J Complement Med*, 2017

Soni, R., et al, "Study on the effect of yoga training on diffusion capacity in chronic obstructive pulmonary disease patients: a controlled trial," *Int J of Yoga*, 2012, Jul–Dec; 5(2), 123–127

Westerdahl, E., "Optimal techniques for deep breathing exercises after cardiac surgery," *Minerva Anesthesiol*, 2015

CDS AND DVDS FOR PRACTICE

Simple Stretches

These exercises can be found on my DVD, Big Yoga Flex-Ability (available at BigYogaOnline.com). Although on the DVD I demonstrate them on the floor, they are easily adapted for the chair.

Relaxation Routines

A free downloadable session can be found on my website, BigYoga Online.com.

Salute to the Sun

A video version of this sequence can be found on my Hatha 1 DVD, available from my website or on Amazon.

Salute to the Sun Using a Chair

A video version of these exercises using a chair can be found on the Big Yoga Flex-Ability DVD.

Restorative Routines

This CD mimics the timing of the routines-download free from website, BigYogaOnline.com.

Progressive Deep Relaxation

This is a recording of instructions for Yogic Sleep. You can download a free audio guide to this practice at www.BigYogaOnline.com.

About the Authors

Meera Patricia Kerr began her study of Yoga in the early 1970s under Sri Swami Satchidananda. After giving birth to her two children, Meera realized that nobody had adapted traditional Yoga poses for the more curvaceous body. As a result, she developed the Big Yoga program, showing people of all shapes and sizes how to enjoy this ancient practice. Meera continues to study and teach Yoga, and is also the best-selling author of *Big Yoga* and *Big Yoga for Less Stress*.

Sandra A. McLanahan, MD, received her medical degree from Wayne State University, and completed a residency in Family Practice at the University of Massachusetts. Dr. McLanahan has served as director of stress management for the Preventive Medicine Research Institute of San Francisco, California. She is currently the founder and Executive Medical Director of Integral Health Services, a holistic health care practice in Buckingham, Virginia. She is a much sought-after speaker in the areas of nutrition, preventive and holistic medicine, and stress management. A long-time student of Integral Yoga, she has been a featured guest on such television programs as *CBS Sunday Morning, NOVA,* and Bill Moyers' *Healing and the Mind* series.

Index

Acupuncture, 32, 71
Aerobic training, 75–76
Alcohol, 45–46
Alveoli, 14
Anti-inflammatory foods, 36
Aromatherapy, 32, 67, 71–72
Asthma, 23–25

Brain, 10
Breathing, act of, 8
Breathing technique
    advanced breathing practices
        cool breath, 155
        hissing breath, 157
        wheezing breath, 156–157
    alternate nostril breathing ,80,
        152–153
    basic
        three-part breath, 93–94
        pursed lip breath, 94
        bellows breath, 150–151
        diaphragmatic breath, 148–149
        humming bee breath, 154–155

Caffeine, 46–48
Cardio-pulmonary resuscitation. *See*
    CPR.
Central nervous system, 11
Chiropractic/osteopathic adjust-
    ments, 72
Chronic bronchitis, 23, 25–26

Chronic obstructive pulmonary dis-
    ease. *See* COPD.
Circulatory system, 17–19
COPD
    asthma, 23–25
    chronic bronchitis, 23, 25–26
    emphysema, 26–27
CPR, 16

Deep relaxation, progressive,
    164–169
Diaphragm, 14–15

Emphysema, 26–27
Epiglottis, 13
Expiratory reserve volume, 22

Fasting, 54–55, 66
Fats, 40–42
Fiber, 39–40
Flex-ability series, 95–96
Functional residual capacity, 22

Garlic, 53

Hair/cilia, nose, 11–12
Heart, 16–17
Herbs
    garlic, 53
    nettles, 53
Hering-breuer reflex, 15, 78

High-intensity interval training.*See*
     HIIT.
HIIT, 76–77
Hyperbaric oxygen treatment, 73

Inflammation
     anti-inflammatory foods, 36
     inflammatory foods, 36
Inflammatory foods, 36
Inspiratory reserve volume, 22

Laughter, 64, 65, 68
Lung disorders, restrictive
     lung removal, partial 29–30
     pneumonia, 28–29
Lung removal, partial 29–30

Lungs
     alveoli, 14
     diaphragm, 14–15
Meditation
     mantra meditation, 161
     so hum meditation, 159–160
Menus, daily, 49–51
Mental activities, stress reduction,
     59–62
Mouth/nasal passages, 11

Nasal dilator strips, 72
Nettles, 53
Non-locomotor exercises, 94–95
Nose
     hair/cilia, 11–12
     nostrils. 12
Nostrils, 12
Nutritional summary, 50–51

Oxygen, 8–10
Oxygen tanks, 72–73

Peak airflow, 22

Physical activities, stress reduction,
     58–59
Phytochemicals, 43
Plant-based diets, 38–39
Pneumonia, 28–29
Practical activities, stress reduction,
     62–65
Props/ clothing, exercise, 86–90
Proteins, 42–43

Residual volume, 22
Resistance to practice, overcoming,
     81–83
Respiratory infections, prevention
     for, 66–71
Respiratory tract, 9
Restorative poses
     heart opener, 141
     hip elevation, 142
     leg elevation, 143–146
     torso opener, 140

Seated sequence, flex-ability series
     ankle circles, 100
     book feet, 99
     chin up, chin down, 113
     ear to shoulder, 115
     elbow bends, 107
     figure eights, 106
     finale, 116–117
     flex and point, 98
     hip juicifier, 102
     knee bends, 101
     love your fingers, 104
     pelvic tilt, 111
     scarecrow, 112
     shoulder squeeze, 103
     side stretch, 109
     side to side, 114
     side twist, 110
     thoracic toning, 108

wrist wrangling, 105

Self-CPR, 16
Simple deep breathing, 78–79
Smoking, how to quit, 31–34
Smoothie, super drink, 48
Standing sequence, flex-ability series
    sun salute at the chair, 127–138
    sun salute at the wall, 119–126
Strength training, 77
Stress reduction
    laughter, 64, 65,68
    mental activities, 59–62
    physical activities, 58–59
    practical activities, 62–64

Sugar, refined, 43–45
Super foods, 40
Supplements
    herbs, 53
    vitamins/minerals, 52–53
Tests, measuring respiratory function
    expiratory reserve volume, 22

functional residual capacity, 22
inspiratory reserve volume, 22
peak airflow, 22
residual volume, 22
tidal volume, 22
total lung capacity, 22
Tidal volume, 22
Tips, exercise, 90–92
Total lung capacity, 22
Treatments, breathing disorders
    acupuncture, 71
    aromatherapy, 71–72
    chiropractic/osteopathic adjustments, 72
    hyperbaric oxygen, 73
    nasal dilator strips, 72
    oxygen tanks, 72–73

Uvula, 13

Visualizations,162–163
Vitamins/minerals, 52–53

Whole foods, 49
Windpipe, 13

Other Square One Titles of Interest

Your Blood Never Lies

How to Read a Blood Test for a Longer, Healthier Life

James B. LaValle, RPh, CCN

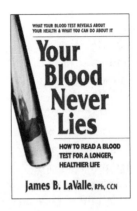

A standard blood test indicates how well the kidneys and liver are functioning, the potential for heart disease, and a host of other vital health markers. Unfortunately, most of us cannot decipher these results ourselves or even formulate the right questions to ask—or we couldn't, until now. *Your Blood Never Lies* clears up the mystery surrounding blood test results. In simple language, Dr. LaValle explains all the information found on these forms, making it understandable and accessible so that you can look at the results yourself and know the significance of each marker.

$16.95 US • 368 pages • 6 x 9-inch paperback • ISBN 978-0-7570-0350-9

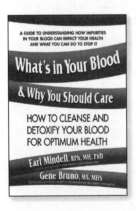

What's In Your Blood & Why You Should Care

How to Cleanse and Detoxify Your Blood for Optimum Health

Earl Mindell, RPh, MH, PhD, and Gene Bruno, Ms, MHS

Like most people, you probably get a blood test and keep your fingers crossed until the results come back. But while these tests focus on key components of your blood, they provide only a limited view of what's going on inside you. Blood tests don't tell you about heavy metals or unwanted pathogens that may be coursing through your body. *What's In Your Blood & Why You Should Care* is the first book to provide a complete picture of the components that make up your blood, how it functions, and what you can do to improve its quality for greater health and longevity. From diets to supplements to medical treatments, it's all there in this groundbreaking book.

$16.95 US • 208 pages • 6 x 9-inch paperback • ISBN 978-0-7570-0443-8

What You Must Know About Vitamins, Minerals, Herbs and So Much More

SECOND EDITION

Choosing the Nutrients That Are Right for You

Pamela Wartian Smith, MD, MPH

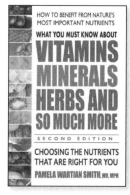

Even if you follow a healthful diet, you are probably not getting all the nutrients you need to prevent disease. Why? There are many reasons, ranging from the mineral-depleted soils in which our foods are grown, to medications that rob the body of various vitamins and minerals. Reflecting the latest scientific research, *What You Must Know About Vitamins, Minerals, Herbs and So Much More—Second Edition* explains how you can restore and maintain health through the wise use of nutrients. Whether you are trying to overcome a medical condition or you simply want to preserve good health, this book will guide you in making the best dietary and supplement choices.

$16.95 US • 512 pages • 6 x 9-inch paperback • ISBN 978-0-7570-0471-1

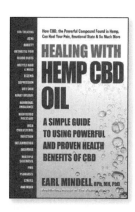

Healing with Hemp CBD Oil

A Simple Guide to Using Powerful and Proven Health Benefits of CBD

Earl Mindell, RPh, MH, PhD

The health benefits of marijuana are now gaining public awareness. Yet hemp—a close relative of marijuana and richer source of CBD (the compound responsible for effectively treating dozens of disorders)—has been classified as a Class 1 drug. For this reason, it cannot be grown commercially in the United States. In *Healing with Hemp CBD Oil,* author Earl Mindell looks at the important role the hemp plant has played in both Eastern and Western societies. After discussing the science behind CBD's medical benefits, he presents an A-to-Z guide of health conditions that can be effectively treated by hemp and CBD oils. *Healing with Hemp CBD Oil* guides you in using this all-natural substance as a remedy that is both safe and side effect free.

$16.95 US • 160 pages • 6 x 9-inch paperback • ISBN 978-0-7570-0455-1

Soft Foods for Easier Eating Cookbook

Easy-to-Follow Recipes for People Who Have
Chewing and Swallowing Problems

Sandra Woodruff, RD, and Leah Gilbert-Henderson, PhD

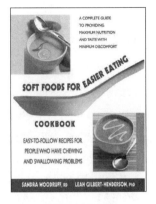

Each year, medical treatments leave millions of patients with chewing and swallowing difficulties. While most hospitals deal with this by puréeing their food, the results are unappetizing. To solve this problem, Sandra Woodruff and Leah Gilbert-Henderson have written *Soft Foods for Easier Eating Cookbook,* an easy-to-follow guide that offers maximum nutrition and taste with minimum discomfort. After presenting simple strategies for living with chewing and swallowing difficulties, the authors provide over 150 recipes for smashing smoothies, sumptuous soups, hearty entrées, and much more.

$18.95 US • 320 pages • 7.5 x 9-inch paperback • ISBN 978-0-7570-0290-8

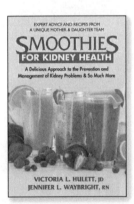

Smoothies for Kidney Health

A Delicious Approach to the Prevention and
Management of Kidney Problems & So Much More

Victoria L. Hulett, JD, and Jennifer L. Waybright, RN

Created by Victoria Hulett, who began losing kidney function at an early age due to an inherited disorder, and her daughter Jennifer Waybright, a registered nurse, *Smoothies for Kidney Health* offers invaluable nutritional information plus easy-to-make smoothie recipes designed to enhance the health of patients at any stage of CKD. After explaining the basics of kidney function, the authors show how certain foods can speed deterioration of kidney function while others can actually safeguard it, preventing or slowing CKD progression. This is followed by eighty kitchen-tested recipes for satisfying smoothies that contain the ingredients scientifically shown to protect kidney health.

$16.95 US • 240 pages • 6 x 9-inch paperback • ISBN 978-0-7570-0411-7

Big Yoga

A Simple Guide for Bigger Bodies

Meera Patricia Kerr

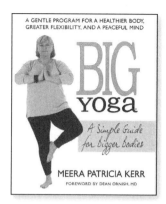

Think yoga is only for skinny young things? Think again. To expert Meera Patricia Kerr, yoga can and should be used by everyone—*especially* plus-size individuals. In *Big Yoga,* Meera shares the unique yoga program she developed for all those who think that yoga is not for them.

Part One of *Big Yoga* begins with a clear explanation of what yoga is, what benefits it offers, and how it can fit into anyone's life. Included is an important discussion of self-image. The book goes on to provide practical information regarding clothing, mats, and suitable environments, and to emphasize the need to begin with care. Part Two offers over forty different exercises specifically designed to work with bigger bodies. In each case, the author explains the technique, details its advantages, and offers step-by-step instructions along with easy-to-follow photographs.

$17.95 US • 240 pages • 7.5 x 9-inch paperback • ISBN 978-0-7570-0215-1

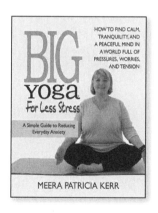

Big Yoga for Less Stress

A Simple Guide to Reducing Everyday Anxiety

Meera Patricia Kerr

We seem to be overwhelmed by stress. We wake up with it, carry it around with us, and even take it to bed. We know we're stressed because we experience the telltale symptoms—tension headaches, nervousness, exhaustion, high blood pressure, and lowered immunity. The truth is that we have the power to control, reduce, and even eliminate the stress we feel. For over thirty-five years, gifted instructor Meera Patricia Kerr has taught thousands of people how to use Yoga to overcome their anxiety and develop greater physical and emotional health. In her new book, *Big Yoga for Less Stress,* Meera provides a complete program of movements and exercises to combat all the stressors in our lives.

$17.95 US • 176 pages • 7.5 x 9-inch paperback • ISBN 978-0-7570-0405-6

The Acid-Alkaline Food Guide
SECOND EDITION

A Quick Reference to Foods &
Their Effect on pH Levels

Dr. Susan E. Brown and Larry Trivieri, Jr.

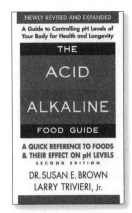

The importance of acid-alkaline balance to good
health is no secret. *The Acid-Alkaline Food
Guide* was designed as an easy-to-follow guide
to the most common foods that influence your
body's pH level. Now in its second edition, this
bestseller has been expanded to include many more domestic
and international foods. Updated information also explores (and
refutes) the myths about pH balance and diet, and guides you to
supplements that can help you achieve a pH level that supports
greater well-being.

$8.95 US • 224 pages • 4 x 7-inch paperback • ISBN 978-0-7570-0393-6

Glycemic Index Food Guide

For Weight Loss, Cardiovascular Health, Diabetic
Management, and Maximum Energy

Dr. Shari Lieberman

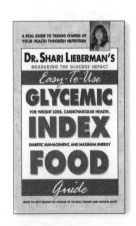

By indicating how quickly a given food triggers
a rise in blood sugar, the glycemic index (GI)
enables you to choose foods that can help you
manage a variety of conditions and improve
your overall health. This easy-to-use guide
teaches you about the GI and how to use it.
It provides both the glycemic index and the
glycemic load for hundreds of foods and beverages, including raw
foods, cooked foods, and many combination and prepared foods.
Whether you want to manage your diabetes, lose weight, increase
your heart health, or simply enhance your well-being, the *Glycemic
Index Food Guide* is the best place to start.

$7.95 US • 160 pages • 4 x 7-inch paperback • ISBN 978-0-7570-0245-8

**For more information on our books,
visit our website at www.squareonepublishers.com**